# The Origin of the Subject in Psychoanalysis

This highly original work uses the Big Bang theory as a conceptual tool to address the question of the origin of the subject in psychoanalysis.

*The Origin of the Subject in Psychoanalysis* elucidates the radical discontinuity between Freud and Lacan in the foundations of their psychoanalytic theories and conceptions of the clinic. Alfredo Eidelsztein argues that just as physics conceives the origin of matter, energy and space-time as an absolute beginning, so the appearance of the symbolic order and the subject must be understood as an "ex-nihilo creation" that excludes any form of causal relationship between the "before" and the "after." He argues that this is a major conceptual difference between Freud and Lacan: the dimension of the signifier, beginning with its appearance, marks an absolute discontinuity from what was before and asserts itself as the condition from which, for the human realm, reality and experience are given. Eidelsztein's conceptions regarding the origin of the subject, the Big Bang of language and speech, and its discontinuity with the biological body establish the basis on which the psychoanalytic clinic should be sustained.

Written in clear and straightforward prose, *The Origin of the Subject in Psychoanalysis* will be of great interest to scholars of Lacanian psychoanalysis and to Lacanian analysts in practice and in training.

**Alfredo Eidelsztein** is an Argentine psychoanalyst. He holds a PhD in psychology from the University of Buenos Aires and is one of the founders and former director of APOLa International. He taught graduate courses at the University of Buenos Aires for more than 30 years and is the author of several books translated into a wide range of languages, including *The Graph of Desire: Using the Work of Jacques Lacan* (Routledge). He is the author of around 200 journal articles published in Spanish, Italian, Portuguese, French, and English, and he teaches internationally. His online seminars can be accessed at www.eidelszteinalfredo.com.ar.

# The Lines of the Symbolic in Psychoanalysis Series

Series Editor:Ian Parker, Manchester Psychoanalytic Matrix

Psychoanalytic clinical and theoretical work is always embedded in specific linguistic and cultural contexts and carries their traces, traces which this series attends to in its focus on multiple contradictory and antagonistic 'lines of the Symbolic'. This series takes its cue from Lacan's psychoanalytic work on three registers of human experience, the Symbolic, the Imaginary and the Real, and employs this distinctive understanding of cultural, communication and embodiment to link with other traditions of cultural, clinical and theoretical practice beyond the Lacanian symbolic universe. The Lines of the Symbolic in Psychoanalysis Series provides a reflexive reworking of theoretical and practical issues, translating psychoanalytic writing from different contexts, grounding that work in the specific histories and politics that provide the conditions of possibility for its descriptions and interventions to function. The series makes connections between different cultural and disciplinary sites in which psychoanalysis operates, questioning the idea that there could be one single correct reading and application of Lacan. Its authors trace their own path, their own line through the Symbolic, situating psychoanalysis in relation to debates which intersect with Lacanian work, explicating it, extending it and challenging it.

**A Social Ontology of Psychosis**
Genea-logical Treatise on Lacan's Conception of Psychosis
*Diego Enrique Londoño-Paredes*

**Ornette Coleman, Psychoanalysis, Discourse**
Movements in Harmolodic Space
*A.L. James*

**The Origin of the Subject in Psychoanalysis**
Rethinking the Foundations of Lacanian Theory and Clinic
*Alfredo Eidelsztein*

For more information about the series, please visit: https://www.routledge.com/The-Lines-of-the-Symbolic-in-Psychoanalysis-Series/book-series/KARNLOS

# The Origin of the Subject in Psychoanalysis

## Rethinking the Foundations of Lacanian Theory and Clinic

Alfredo Eidelsztein

Translated By Nicolás Garrera-Tolbert

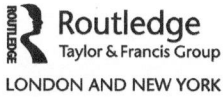
Routledge
Taylor & Francis Group

LONDON AND NEW YORK

Designed cover image: "El eslabón perdido" ["The Missing Link"], by Alfredo Eidelsztein, cedar sculpture, 20x26x10cm, Buenos Aires, 2004

First English edition published 2025
by Routledge
4 Park Square, Milton Park, Abingdon, Oxon, OX14 4RN

and by Routledge
605 Third Avenue, New York, NY 10158

*Routledge is an imprint of the Taylor & Francis Group, an informa business*

© 2025 Alfredo Eidelsztein

The right of Alfredo Eidelsztein to be identified as author[/s] of this work has been asserted in accordance with sections 77 and 78 of the Copyright, Designs and Patents Act 1988.

First Spanish edition published by Letra Viva 2021

First English edition published by Routledge 2025

Translated by Nicolás Garrera-Tolbert

*British Library Cataloguing-in-Publication Data*
A catalogue record for this book is available from the British Library

ISBN: 978-1-032-77905-8 (hbk)
ISBN: 978-1-032-77904-1 (pbk)
ISBN: 978-1-003-48533-9 (ebk)

DOI: 10.4324/9781003485339

Typeset in Times New Roman
by codeMantra

# Contents

**PART IV**
**Appendix** 99

# Foreword

*Nicolás Garrera-Tolbert*

A remarkable feature of Jacques Lacan's psychoanalytic theory is its anti-naturalism: a frontal rejection of any attempt to think of the human in continuity with animality, that is, a domain in which being and living happens outside the universal, omnipresent medium of discourse. This anti-naturalistic trait, developed to its ultimate logical consequences, that is, thematized as a thesis and elucidated as a concept, is sufficient to establish *a rupture, at the level of the epistemic, ethical, and ontological foundations, of Lacanian theory with respect to that of Freud, the post-Freudians, Freudo-Lacanism, and all the attempts to inscribe psychoanalysis in the so-called "life sciences,"* particularly through the developments of neuroscience. Indeed, the anti-naturalistic feature of Lacanian theory is a direct consequence of what Alfredo Eidelsztein considers to be at the heart of this theory, namely, Lacan's theory of the subject, which can be formally characterized as follows: *the object of psychoanalysis—that which psychoanalysis produces as its field of study and, correlatively, of psychoanalytic experience—is the subject: a discursive reality created by the analyst as a complex articulation of signifiers, whose meaning is elucidated by an analytical, speculative (but not arbitrary) operation that writes this subject as a text.* If the subject is rigorously conceived as a new and particular genre of discourse,[1] fundamental psychoanalytic concepts will have to be re-examined, no matter how well established they seem to be, exclusively within this frame. Thus, in this view, the subject does *not* pre-exist its production in analysis, "*the* unconscious" is *not* an intrinsic or transhistorical feature of "the mind," and the analytic "attitude" does *not* consist in an attentive, free-floating listening stance out of which a supposedly adequate (but ultimately unjustifiable) interpretation will arise. In particular, the regime of affectivity and the alleged *bodily* drives are conceived by Lacan as *effects of the signifying order*. As such, their intelligibility is revealed through an analytical interpretation of a highly specific nature, which inevitably reflects the analyst's theoretical commitments. The opposition between Freud and Lacan on these key issues of psychoanalytic theory and practice is maximal.

Eidelsztein goes even further. Indeed, he shows that if the subject is entirely an effect of discourse, a phenomenon of language, then the notions of freedom, subjective responsibility, and *jouissance* have no role to play in psychoanalysis.[2]

Moreover, the psychoanalytic subject so construed has no body, no sex, no organs, and no brain: it is no longer a psycho-physical individual.[3] Accordingly, Eidelsztein's conception of the cure bets everything on the possibility of reconfiguring the particular (not singular, *nota bene*) subject of each case. Such reconfiguration coincides with the creation of a *new* subject. Thus, by unfolding the far-reaching logical and clinical consequences of the *"Ur-Faktum"* [the original, primordial, brute fact] of the primacy of the signifier in the speculative creation of the subject, Eidelsztein proposes an anti-individualistic, anti-substantialist, and anti-nihilist psychoanalysis.[4]

Although it can be read as an autonomous text, *Freud Should Not Be Saved* is in strict continuity with Eidelsztein's *Another Lacan: A Critical Study of the Foundations of Lacanian Psychoanalysis* (2015). The latter, not yet translated into English, examines the reasons for the Lacanian questioning of the ontotheological tradition, that is, the foundations of the West's philosophical project as articulating itself starting from the postulation of substance as the determining model or paradigm of being. Simplifying things dramatically, one could claim that in this tradition, something properly is if and only if: (i) *it is identical to itself*: something is *one* when it remains identical to itself through its always partial modifications, (ii) *it is self-subsistent*: something self-subsists when its identity lies solely within itself and (iii) *it plays the role of logical and ontological foundation*. To this model, Eidelsztein opposes Lacan's "hontology" (*hontologie*: in French, this is a neologism [*honte* {shame, disgrace} + *ontologie*]) which posits a *subject-without-substance*, never self-subsisting, inevitably contingent, only imaginarily one, in a necessary relation to the symbolic orders that engendered it, and, consequently, susceptible to being transfigured at its root through symbolic interventions. The transformative power of psychoanalysis is thus reaffirmed and rationally justified within a new, non-Freudian ontological framework.

The longest and most important essay in this book, *The Origin of the Subject in Psychoanalysis* (2012), addresses a problem that *Another Lacan* left unexamined. Its crucial claim is that the origin of the subject is an ex-nihilo creation (like the physical universe according to the Big Bang Theory), the existence of which owes nothing to the natural domain. For Eidelsztein, between the natural and the signifying realm there is an unfulfillable, absolute gap. In the specific field of human affairs, the signifier—always open, in principle, to a new interpretation—is the ultimate ground of the human, but, given the signifier's logic, it is *Grund* as well as *Abgrund*, both foundation and abyss of the human. In line with what Foucault referred to as characteristic of philosophy, psychoanalysis practiced on this basis is the work of incessant questioning, always restarted, of how we (each particular subject) actually think, exist, and live. That is, it questions *the field of the possible and the impossible in each case* (the latter constituting perhaps an eminent definition of "subject"), to think, be, and live in another way, one that tempers or eliminates useless suffering and enhances the value of living in such a way that one can affirm him/her/their self while remaining integrally open, permeated, and nourished by the Other and the others.[5]

Lacan's project made explicit, restarted, invigorated, and continued by Eidelsztein and by the members of the institution he founded is today more radical than ever.[6] It stands against contemporary naturalism, nihilism, individualism, and cynicism.[7] It is from the absolute onto-epistemic primacy of the signifier that a new psychoanalysis offers a way out of the contemporary reification and animalization of the human (something conducive to fundamentally racist and discriminatory social and political practices). Eidelsztein's psychoanalysis is also an effective challenge to post-truth ideologies and even a salient counterpoint to the most recent, wild forms of scientism. The ultimate indeterminacy of the signifier does not make truth impossible. Quite the opposite: truth is an intrinsically signifying matter and, as such, is open to history and the future. It allows, on the plane of what is abstractly meant by the names "individual" and "collective," that life can be something other than what, for better or worse, it has become in our day. *This* psychoanalysis, so understood, wants to be a genuinely transformative practice.

Nicolás Garrera-Tolbert, PhD, LP
www.drnicolasgarreratolbert.com
New York City
April 2024

## Notes

1  Cf. Montesano, Haydée, *El texto clínico: Un nuevo género de discurso* (Buenos Aires: Letra Viva, 2021).
2  *Jouissance* in Miller's sense, (not Lacan's), i.e., a *jouissance* that is reified, substantialized, irreducibly individual, singular, and therefore ultimately ineffable, unalterable, and therapeutically unapproachable.
3  For the theoretical and clinical implications of this thesis, see, in this volume, "Sex, Gender, and Sexuality in Lacanian Perspective," pp. 92 For Eidelsztein's account of the psychoanalytic body, see his *No hay substancia corporal. Controversias sobre el cuerpo, la sociedad, y el psicoanálisis* (Buenos Aires: Letra Viva, 2023).
4  See his *Otro Lacan. Estudio crítico sobre los fundamentos filosóficos del psicoanálisis lacaniano* (Buenos Aires: Letra Viva, 2015).
5  Very schematically, one may say that, responding to the challenge of contemporary nihilism, in and out of psychoanalysis, Eidelsztein's original reading of *objet a* conceptualizes it as that which, being valued, is capable of orienting our existence in the direction of an accretion of life in ourselves.
6  APOLa: Asociación para Otro Lacan [in Spanish]: http://apola.online/
7  APOLa's Research Program is articulated around these contemporary modalities of human suffering. Its conception of psychoanalysis aims to give itself the means for therapeutic action on the symptoms caused by these forms of subjective suffering. The Program can be found here: https://apola.online/programa.

# Series Preface for Afredo Eidelsztein's *The Origin of the Subject in Psychoanalysis: Rethinking the Foundations of Lacanian Theory and Clinic*

This extraordinary book revolves around a series of ineliminable gaps in psycho-analytic theory and clinical practice. These are gaps we need to attend to if we are to grasp both what was revolutionary about Freud's naturalistic conception of the human subject, a human being tragically grounded in and unable to escape its animal nature, and what was revolutionary about Lacan's break from Freud, a break that was announced as a "return" but which gave us something quite new.

To speak of an "origin" of the subject must, according to Alfredo Eidelsztein in this painstaking reconstruction of the trajectory of Lacan away from Freud, also contend with developmentalist and naturalistic origin stories. These stories give us a convenient narrative through which we are able to trace the elaboration of a Lacanian psychoanalysis from its Freudian beginnings that is then, it is often said (by Lacanians) still authentically Freudian, and, in the realm of the clinic, these stories house various developmental narratives by which we can stitch together an account of why we are who we are with reference to where we came from and what happened to us.

Such stories are surely "imaginary," fictive accounts of the history of psychoanalysis and of each personal history, that smooth over contradictions and comfort us. In that way too, the realm of the symbolic is itself susceptible to imaginarization, and, instead of being the ground of being, the symbolic is turned into a set of self-replicating mirrored-wall rooms in a self-satisfying maze of our own making.

The foundations of the Lacanian clinic, in contrast, lie in ruptures, gaps. What Lacan enables is a rupture with Freud that is also indebted to what Freud opened up for us, and this book works away at the theoretical and clinical consequences of that rupture so that we confront not only the origin of Lacan's conception of the subject, but the origin of the human subject as such. Now we are in the domain of the real, and of a conception of the subject as founding itself as if ex nihilo, a moment of conception that is as if the correlate of the "big bang" of the universe that inaugurates being and, at the very same moment, shatters it, pulls away the ground we usually appeal to, that we usually assume to provide a normative origin story.

Psychoanalytic clinical and theoretical work circulates through multiple inter-secting antagonistic symbolic universes. This series opens connections between different cultural sites in which Lacanian work has developed in distinctive ways, in forms of work that question the idea that there could be single correct reading and application. The Lines of the Symbolic in Psychoanalysis series provides a reflexive reworking of psychoanalysis that transmits Lacanian writing from around the world, steering a course between the temptations of a metalanguage and imaginary reduction, between the claim to provide a god's eye view of psychoanalysis and the idea that psychoanalysis must everywhere be the same. And the elaboration of psychoanalysis in the symbolic here grounds its theory and practice in the history and politics of the work in a variety of interventions that touch the real.

Ian Parker
Manchester Psychoanalytic Matrix

# Part I

# Overture

# Chapter 1

# Freud Should Not Be Saved

I cannot evade the notion (though I hesitate to give it expression) that for women the level of what is ethically normal is different from what it is in men. Their super-ego is never so inexorable, so impersonal, so independent of its emotional origins as we require it to be in men.[1]

(S. Freud, 1925)

In its already relatively extensive history, psychoanalysis has confronted criticisms and objections, both real and imaginary, coming from very different sources, among which include the following: Victorian morality, Left-wing movements (which may be surprising), psychiatry, both short-term therapies (of course, here "short" is opposed to the "long duration" of psychoanalytic treatments) as well as CBT, neuroscience, and, finally, feminism and gender and queer studies. With the exception of Lacan, after Freud's death, the strategy implemented by psychoanalysts to barricade themselves against criticism (let us not forget that psychoanalysis is the therapeutic practice that has received the most violent, systematic, virulent, and ruthless attacks) consisted of withdrawing into themselves, closing ranks, and pretending that those criticisms did not exist. Thus, psychoanalysis embraced a dangerous "ostrich policy" and as a consequence enabled the spreading of inadmissible and unjustified arguments. Much worse, it deprived itself of "receiving its own message in an inverted form from the Other" (Lacan), the optimal way to prevent falling into stubbornness and mental obstruction by leaving open and making prosperous the "way of truth." The explicit argumentative basis that psychoanalysts used to sustain such a policy was the allegedly legitimate application of the following reasoning: psychoanalysis can be justified or criticized solely from within (incidentally, neither of these have happened yet). It is believed that its knowledge and practice emerge from itself and that no outsider has the right to critique it. It is claimed that the psychoanalyst learns from his own practice and that what the latter cannot teach he can obtain from his own personal analysis. Thus, if anything is criticized or misunderstood about psychoanalysis, it will immediately be dismissed by the psychoanalyst as the judgment of someone who is unqualified to yield it for not having made enough progress in his personal analysis or for

DOI: 10.4324/9781003485339-2

lacking clinical experience. This procedure of self-validation was diagnosed by Jean-Marie Vaysse as a self-creation [fundación] myth.[2]

In my view, the systematic application of this myth as a form of ignoring, repressing, and refuting criticism has had two serious consequences. First, such a strategy made it impossible to consider the multiple sources of Freud's theoretical model in a systematic manner, i.e., it became impossible to acknowledge the ungrounded and genuinely contradictory character of his argument (psychoanalysis was born out of the practice of psychoanalysis) and to evaluate the relevance of those sources. Below I offer a partial list of those concepts in Freud's theory whose sources were identified by Freud himself. This list will give the reader a clear sense of how extensively psychoanalysis integrated concepts that belonged to other disciplines and domains of knowledge. Naturally, I do not deny that Freud was the exclusive creator of psychoanalysis as a practice and as a theoretical discipline, which was both absolutely new, and which made possible in the West the reflection on certain aspects of the subject entirely unknown before Freud.

| Concept Integrated to Psychoanalysis by Freud | Source |
| --- | --- |
| Mnemic images | Carl Wernicke |
| Libido | Richard von Krafft-Ebing |
| Autoerotism | Havelock Ellis |
| Bisexuality | Wilhelm Fliess |
| Infantile sexuality | Albert Moll |
| Erogenous zones | Iwan Bloch |
| The opposition between representations and drives [pulsiones] | Arthur Schopenhauer |
| Economic theory of hysterical attacks | Josef Breuer |
| Psychic forces of attraction and repulsion | Ernst Brücke |
| Principle of constancy | Gustav Theodor Fechner |
| The unconscious as "other scene" | Gustav Theodor Fechner |
| The uncanny | Friedrich Schelling |
| The id | Georg Groddeck |
| The indiciary paradigm | Giovanni Morelli |
| Ambivalence | Eugen Bleuler |
| Introversion | Karl Gustav Jung |
| Paternal imago | Karl Gustav Jung |
| Inertia principle | Isaac Newton |
| Parapraxis | Hans Gross |
| The omnipotence of thought | Jean-Baptiste Lamarck |

The second consequence of the self-creation myth, the one that makes so many critics of psychoanalysis claim that psychoanalysts maintain as a rule an almost religious adherence to Freud's theory, is that it generated the notion of an omniscient Freud, i.e., the notion that Freud already knew everything that psychoanalysis could possibly become, even, for instance, everything that Lacan would later create as a new theoretical model half a century later. There are even those who believe that all of Freud's mistakes were caught and rectified by Freud himself. Thus, Freud is perhaps the last figure in the West (it seems that Marx no longer belongs to this group) still posited as a genius possessing eternal and entirely true knowledge.

However, we have been in a radically new situation for many years. In the West, the estimation and position of "women" has changed significantly. This change consists not only of what has been theorized by feminism and gender studies, but has also reached broad layers of the Western population and is a component of prevailing views among younger generations. Further, it is now a fundamental issue in progressive politics. For large sections of the Western population, Freud's work is frankly unacceptable and, in many cases, humiliating and degrading. The kind of criticism that gender studies and feminism have been leveling at Freud for half a century has now passed into "common sense" for the most progressive sectors of the population. And yet, psychoanalysts, for the most part, are not willing to listen to, consider, or accept them.

Let us consider it briefly here: for Freud, the material and scientific basis on which psychoanalysis is based is biology. This is why he always considered psychoanalysis to be scientific while his critics, from Karl Popper to Mario Bunge, were indignant against it. On the other hand, for Lacan, the basis of psychoanalysis is provided by logic, linguistics, mathematical-physics, and topology.[3] The set of all these disciplines (including psychoanalysis) is what Lacan proposes to designate as the field of "conjectural sciences:" they operate through the mathème, with purely abstract entities, and under the hypothetical-deductive method.

By grounding his theory in biology and adhering to a strongly inductivist model, Freud derives: (a) the life and death drives from inherent properties of the living substance, (b) gender positions from anatomical sex, and (c) the Oedipus complex from the natural conditions under which children are raised by female mothers and male fathers. On this basis, he even goes so far as to consider homosexuality a disturbance of psychosexual development. Regardless of what can be said about his personal commitment to misogyny, patriarchy, Eurocentrism, and sexism—which I will not discuss here—it is unquestionable that Freud ends up developing a psychoanalysis that is organized around anatomical sexual differences determined at the time of birth and the biological destiny of each individual, which enabled sexist prejudices to endure within his theory. Quite the opposite, for Lacan, "father," "mother," "woman," and the like are signifying constructs.

In my view, the core of the problem is that, although in modern Western society—at least in its less atavistic, conservative, and religious sectors—such conceptions have already been overcome, in psychoanalysis they have not. One's place in culture, sexuality, economics, politics, knowledge, power, family, etc., absolutely depends on linguistic, historical, ideological, sociological, and cultural conditions. The same applies to conceptions of biology and anatomy: they are intertwined and ultimately contingent on those conditions.

Thus, in our time and culture, it is simply unacceptable to sustain claims such as: women envy men's penises, women's moral and ethical (i.e., superegoic) capacities are lesser than those of men, the personal fulfillment of women can only be attained by their becoming biological mothers, and the psychosexual position of children is equivalent to that of peoples considered to be primitive. All this should be publicly acknowledged by psychoanalysts involved in the modern debate. One effect of dispensing with Freud's arguments is the possibility of taking full advantage of the power of Lacan's formulations. Lacan substitutes Freud's biological mother for the Mother's Desire as the embodiment of the Other, i.e., a function that can be performed by a heterosexual couple, a woman or two, a man or two, or an institution, to name some examples. Further, through his notion of paternal metaphor, Lacan substitutes Freud's male father for the Name-of-the-Father, a function that should not be embodied by anyone and that operates by inscribing the impotence of the Other. Finally, Lacan substitutes the son for a third term, resulting from the operation of the Father's metaphor, which does not entail the intervention of anything biological, pre-determined, or teleological.

In the face of the crucial challenge our time poses to psychoanalysis, it is not enough to omit Freud's claims, to say nothing about them, to pretend they were never said, or to claim that if they were said it was due to Freud's being a child of his own time. It is necessary to sustain a systematic, rational, and explicit critique of these pseudo-scientistic arguments, such that we might rewrite the whole theoretical model of psychoanalysis under an absolutely different logic in open debate with all the disciplines with which it coexists. Lacan tried to do this, but, due to the hegemony of the irrational defense of the Freudian model among psychoanalysts, he failed, as he himself acknowledged on more than a dozen occasions.[4]

The attempt to "save Freud," along with his unacceptable conceptions, not only fails to contribute to the existence and future development of psychoanalysis, but may also entail the danger of leaving it without a future, since it would close the doors to young people, who are already quite convinced that at the basis of sexual difference as sustained in Freud's work, there lies a chauvinist prejudice. In spite of what is assumed among psychoanalysts, the conditions of possibility of a future for psychoanalysis as a discourse, practice, and theoretical model do not lie in the old heirs of the Freudian legacy, but among younger generations of psychoanalysts. It is not a question of "return" but of "progress."

If psychoanalysis affiliates with a program consisting in subverting the subject, it must itself be entirely open to being subverted at its foundations, just as modern scientific practices (unlike religious and political ones) are. This urgently requires that psychoanalysis give up its defense of Freud, an author who does not require such a defense, since he is indelibly inscribed in the group of thinkers who were and are fundamental in the history of humanity for the conception of the subject. It is precisely for this reason that it is necessary to drop what is "clearly obsolete in the work of a peerless master."[5] "What is obvious is that women lack nothing."[6]

## Notes

1 Freud, Sigmund, "Some Psychical Consequences of the Anatomical Distinction between the Sexes," in the *Standard Edition*, vol. XIX, 1925, pp. 257–58.
2 Vaysse, Jean-Marie, *L'inconscient des modernes. Essai su l'origine métaphysique de la psychanalyse* (Paris: Gallimard, 1999).
3 I have analyzed this issue extensively in my *Segundo Seminario Internacional*: "Lacan: la crítica a Freud desde el psicoanálisis." The seminar is available online here: https://fliphtml5.com/frpt/gzur/Lacan%2C_la_cr%C3%ADtica_a_Freud_desde_el_psicoan%C3%A1lisis/ (last accessed: October 22, 2023).
4 Eidelsztein, Alfredo, "El fracaso de Lacan," in *El rey está desnudo, Issues 2 and 3* (Buenos Aires: Letra Viva, 2009 and 2010).
5 See "The Psychical Effects of the Imaginary Mode," section three of Lacan's "Presentation on Psychic Causality," in *Écrits* (New York: Norton, 2006), p. 146/179.
6 Lacan, Jacques, *Seminar X* (New York: Polity, 2014). Session of March 13, 1963. *Staferla*, p. 119.

# Part II

# Theoretical Perspectives

Chapter 2

# The Concept of Subject in Lacan's Theory[1]

The concept of subject [Fr. *sujet*] could well be the fundamental feature of Western philosophy—or even philosophy *tout court*. It is also one of the main threads in Jacques Lacan's psychoanalytic theory. As the problem of the *origin* of the subject in Lacanian theory is one of the main topics of this book, it would be useful to make clear from the start what I take to be the core meaning of the *Lacanian* subject (hereafter, simply "subject"). Thus, what follows is a sketch of such concept of the subject, which aims to situate it as a problem for psychoanalysis.

## The Meanings of Subject

Let us begin by distinguishing among five different meanings of subject, each referring to a particular domain: linguistics, anthropology, grammar, philosophy, and Lacan's theory.

In psychoanalysis, the concept of subject was first introduced by Lacan. Lacan's use of the term subject is identical to its use in colloquial French: referring to issue, topic, or subject-matter (cf. the *Grand Robert Dictionary of French language*). This is also the ordinary meaning of the term subject in English.

Second, there is its anthropological meaning: it may be considered as an anthropological universal, i.e., when anthropologists refer to the object of their study as a whole, each unit of this whole is called a subject. Not long ago, instead of subject, one would have used the term man. In fact, this is what "anthropology" means, namely, the study, the theory of man. Fortunately, as a consequence of the growth of the feminist movement, we were compelled to change this language, and now, instead of saying, "the study of men and women," we generally use the term subject. According to this usage, each of us is a subject. But this is precisely the problem with this view, namely, that especially in the West, modern man is conceived as identical to the "individual."[2] This is also a problem for psychoanalysis because psychology and the Freudian psychoanalytic tradition—not Lacan's theory—still operate within such conception and therefore contribute to reinforce these individualistic tendencies. This confusion is so pervasive that it is difficult to imagine what "subject" would mean if anything other than "individual."

DOI: 10.4324/9781003485339-4

Consider, however, the Montagues and the Capulets of *Romeo and Juliet*. There was a time where it was entirely acceptable that when any member of group A killed a member of group B, any member of group B automatically held the right to kill any member of group A (and vice versa). For us, immersed as we are in an individualistic logic, such a way of proceeding is unjustifiable. Moreover, according to this logic, the sole author of a crime is the individual who performed the act and not, say, any member of his or her family. Actually, our legal systems, highly individualistic in their ways of functioning, operate according to this logic. On the contrary, cartels and urban gangs are permeated by a different logic—the logic of groups. This is precisely why they are called "cartels" or "gangs" they do not work according to the logic of individualism. So, if I am part of a cartel or tribe, I take the killing of any member as if I had been the target. As seen in many mafia movies, when a goodfella attempts to leave the family, he ends up paying with his life. The prevailing logic is definitely *not* an individualistic one.

The same point can be illustrated differently. I once had a conversation with a person who works at a tourist complex at the Iguazú Waterfalls in Argentina. He told me that although he was born to be a hunter, he had no choice but to become a tour guide, for there were no animals in the area. There is no particular desire that belongs to him. In many tribes around the globe, men hunt and fish, while women raise the children and build up the tents and keep them clean. The question, "What would you like to be when you grow up?" is absent. The role of each member is socially established. My claim is not, however, that the individual pole is entirely absent. After all, one may want to become a shaman, another the leader of the tribe, and yet another one a tourist guide. Interestingly enough, he mentioned that there was a time where all the tents were concentrated in the same area, whereas now they tend to be scattered, spread out. Here we can observe, once again, the preponderance of the individualistic logic.

Let us notice that although subject, as an anthropological universal, has become a synonym for individual, the latter is usually regarded as an epiphenomenon of the biological body. If a man, an individual, is indeed one, what gives consistency to this "one" is thought to be the biological body. Thus, when we want to know, say, how many students are in a classroom, we proceed by counting their bodies. We are entirely convinced that each of them is a subject. But if a student spends the class sleeping or playing with his phone, is he really present? Clearly, the question may be raised as to whether the mere fact that their bodies are present entails that they are genuinely present. In this epoch, the foundation of presence is assumed to be the anatomical body.

The third meaning of subject that must be considered is the subject-predicate relation. In this case, a subject is the object of speech, for instance, a family, a socio-economic class, or a country. A sentence such as, "They will never give up; they will fight until the end" may refer to a people, a group of countries, or a sports team.

The fourth meaning is the philosophical one. Here one must take into account the etymology of "subject," which sends us back to the Aristotelian "*hypokéimenon,*" translated to Latin as "*subjectum*." In this sense, "subject" means what is placed underneath and operates as foundation or grounding. Lacan unequivocally rejects this idea of subject as substance, challenging that a subject can be conceived as a sort of kernel of identity that would remain identical to itself over time, securing thereby its perdurability. It is worth noticing that the philosophical tradition that thinks of subject as *hypokéimenon* stems from the philosophical theory of argumentation, also criticized by Lacan, that holds that "subject" is that which lies behind and operates as the presupposition of what is asserted or argued for.

## Lacan's Concept of Subject

### Against Individualism in Psychoanalytic Theory

The fifth meaning to be considered is Lacan's *new* concept of subject.[3] Although it stands separate from the linguistic, anthropological, grammatical, and philosophical notions of subject, this conception is not intrinsically psychoanalytic. In fact, if it were better known, it could become a useful concept in philosophy and anthropology.

In his 1966 Baltimore presentation, given in the context of a conference on structuralism, Lacan argues that the positing of a structure is necessary for any consideration of the subject and characterizes this structure as an inmixing of alterity. An inmixing is a mix whose elements are no longer distinguishable; it is a synonym for "blended." For instance, if I throw some pen-ink to my coffee, I won't be able to separate the components. Thus, for Lacan, any thought of the subject must be structural in nature: it requires the positing of a structure. Further, in this structure, the subject is blended, indistinguishable from the Other.

Let us be clear: none of this will be found in Freud. For him, there is no meaning for the subject. The differences between Freud and Lacan can be visualized as follows:

| Freud | Lacan |
|---|---|
| Representation | Signifier |
| Oedipal complex | Paternal metaphor |
| Psychic individual | Subject |

According to Freud, the psychic individual, universally considered, is the conflictive product of the encounter of biological energies, the drives, which constitute the *id*; the super-ego, which denotes, for Freud, the moral baggage we are all born with; and society and culture as represented by the ego. The Oedipal plot is the scene and setting of this conflict. It is therefore a conflict between the id, the super-ego, and society and culture. This universal confrontation takes place in each of us and, as a consequence, the individual always suffers from an internal split, which is our universal condition as humans, even when the splitting does not ultimately alter our unity. It is a splitting that does not happen at any level of animal life, for no animal is invested by society and culture as something internal to it. After the dissolution [*sepultamiento*][4] of the Oedipal plot, the splitting becomes permanent. The resolution of the struggle among the passions, drives, the social, and the cultural determines what the individual, as a subject of a society, will be: a murderer, a pervert, a saint, a homosexual, a good parent, etc.

The idea of a division of psychic personality is not only an idea of Freud's, but a product of culture. One finds it, for instance, in Stevenson's 1886 novel, *The Strange Case of Dr. Jekyll and Mr. Hyde*. I don't think Freud ever quoted it, but the characters are Freudian in nature. Dr. Jekyll and Mr. Hyde became immensely popular at that time. Another eminent example of this is Herman Hesse's 1928, *Steppenwolf*. Today we would perhaps think of The Hulk. He is a theoretical physicist, a true gentleman, but when he loses it, he becomes a monster. For many, Dr. Jekyll is a representative of alcoholism, someone who drinks heavily at night and, as a result, becomes a monster. Either way, all of them are examples of a split in the psychic personality. Even today, many of our patients present their psychic economy by reference to such a dynamic: "I keep playing it cool, swallowing it all over and over…until I'm fed up and can't take it any more and then I explode." It is the same logic. Patients often make use of this levee's logic: they hold it in until they totally lose it. At first sight, one may be tempted to think of Jack Moore, the main character of David Fincher's 1999 film, *Fight Club*, as a contemporary example of Jekyll/Hyde. In my view, though, splitting and confrontation, in the movie, are not presented as parts of his personality; I take it as a case of psychosis.

As it has been maintained by several scholars, Freud took modern individualism to an extreme. His "psychological" theory holds the notion that we all live in an internal world—the extension of which coincides, precisely, with the limits of our individuality—that is intrinsically conflictive. Remo Bodei illustrates this Freudian conviction with the notion of "the soul's nerves." And Norbert Elias, to my mind the best scholar on individuation processes (an author poorly known in his lifetime and never quoted by Lacan), suggests that that our society is going through a time when its components are thought of as individuals—just as we think of ourselves. He may have been the first to advance the model that our society can be seen as a billiard table where individuals are like balls bumping against each other.[5]

For Freud, living in a culture entails discontent. This is because we are born with drives that, due to the presence of civilization, cannot be satisfied in a direct and fulfilling manner. As a result, our interests are always in conflict and their realization delayed. Thus, we are bumping against each other and each of us against society. But there is no necessity in this view. Actually, let us recall that Schrödinger, who, already since 1938, argued that neither atoms nor their electrons are little balls. In our schools, however, it is still generally taught that the electron goes around the nucleus as the earth goes around the sun. Quantum physics challenges the notion that subatomic matter is made of corpuscles.

The corpuscular model is the same as Freud's, as his representation for the psychic individual is an egg (see next page). To this model, Lacan opposes the torus, which can be seen as a pierced egg with a hole at its center. This is why it is important to study topology. The torus is an egg turned into a ring, a pierced egg: one could put a finger or even another torus through it. If the latter, each torus' heart would be traversed by the other torus (see below).

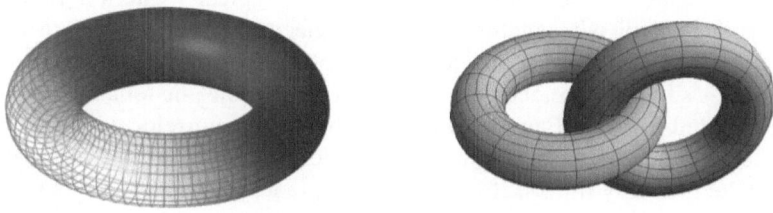

According to Freud, interhuman relationships could be conceived of according to the following diagram:

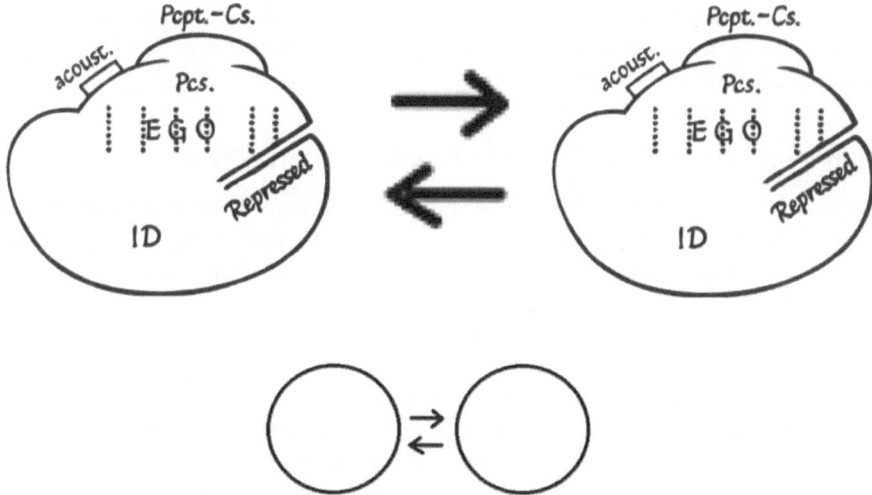

In the West, social functioning goes hand in hand with the Freudian model. Other people, in their strivings, are opposed to me and my own strivings. Thus, forming a family, having children, and maintaining a relationship have become less and less frequent. It is assumed that the precondition to be in a relationship is to give up what one wants. This is our modern condition. Earlier, instead of asking, "Where do I want to go?" one would have asked, "Where are we going?" This is why we see an increasing number of single-person households.

In rich countries, there are more people living alone than people living with others. Obviously, I'm assuming that "living alone" refers to a situation where there is only one human living in that household—obviously, there may also be a dog, a cat, or a snake (incidentally, many people today have a very intense affective relationship with their pets). Certainly, Freud did not create this situation and is not responsible for it. However, his conceptions point in this direction: "I satisfy myself in my own person and I identify with myself only when I distinguish myself and distance myself from others." This is a typical Western notion. Consider: a young person whose father and grandfather are lawyers decides to seek an interview with a vocational counselor. He is looking for advice on his career path because he is somewhat undecided. After several sessions, he tells the counselor that he decided to study Law. How do you think the counselor will react? It is most likely that he feels disappointed and invites him to reexamine his decision. After all, he probably thinks, if his father and grandfather are both lawyers, his decision may not be *his own*. If the young man had communicated, instead, that his decision was to study the oboe, the counselor would have probably finalized the interviews and encouraged him to embrace his passion and become a member of the local symphonic orchestra. Now consider, in contrast, the tribe where men will be hunters like their fathers and grandfathers before them. The difference is noteworthy. In sum, that we think of desire as fundamentally individual is a feature of our society and culture. This has not always been the case, and it does not have to be the case now. Consequently, not realizing one's individual desire does not need to cause any frustration.

### Against Representationalism in Psychoanalytic Theory

As anticipated, Lacan's subject must primarily be considered equivalent to the topic, issue, and subject-matter. Evidence of this is that Lacan, having already coined the notion of the subject from the very beginning of his teaching and never abandoning it, creates the figure of the analysand. Freud created the figure of the analyst and Lacan that of the analysand. These figures do not dilute the notion of subject. Indeed, the subject is the topic, issue, or subject-matter elaborated by both analyst and analysand. Lacan conceives of this subject from a minimal formula. It is actually the simplest of his formulas: a subject is what a signifier represents for another signifier. This is an argumentative principle attempting to abandon Freud's mnemic trace and, correlatively, the individualism entailed by it.

Indeed, with his theory of representation, Freud nurtures the West's individualistic tendencies. Think, for instance, of his notion of mnemic trace, which he understands as the individual mark left by the particular lived experiences [*vivencias*] one goes through. The mnemic trace works as an internal duplicate of an event that affects an individual. "Thing-representations," which for Freud are the primary psychical representations and constitute the nucleus of the unconscious, operate for us as the thing itself. This is why Freud claims that desiring ends up in hallucinating, for carrying the trace is the equivalent of being again in the presence of the object. "Word-representations" are also marks in the psychic apparatus—in this case, the apparatus of someone having registered something through speech.

Lacan's formula of the subject establishes that there are no longer traces of any object or lived experiences that are intrinsically personal. To elaborate a topic, issue, or subject-matter, at least two signifiers are needed. This follows from Saussure's theory of the signifier: a signifier, taken in isolation, in itself, does not mean anything. It follows that it could hardly be the trace of anything. If a signifier meant what it allegedly means according to the dictionary, one should admit as a tautology that, say, "cow" means cow. Lacan's theory has nothing to do with it. Indeed, the topic/issue/subject-matter is elaborated through signifiers, but only within the system of their mutual relations in the structure of language and always in a particular discursive context, for instance, a psychoanalytic one. Consider: a patient tells us he is depressed; we write down "depression." Next, we ask him why he is feeling that way and he responds that he has been fired and no longer has a job. Now, we write down "job." For Lacan, we should take these terms as signifiers, i.e., as not signifying anything in and of themselves: *what they mean must be determined—this is precisely our task as analysts—only on the basis of an analysis of the particular contexts in which those signifiers, in virtue of their mutual relations, begin to signify*. We always proceed in a conjectural manner. Other discursive contexts will avail or discredit our conjecture. For instance, it may well be the case that in the context of this patient's family history "depression" and "job" are articulated with "money" and "divorce."

From the same theory of the signifier, it follows that there is no signifier that identifies the subject. This is why a subject cannot be either a person or even a split individual: it is a topic, an issue that must be conceived as what is represented among signifiers and also in-between analyst and analysand. The latter is the discursive dimension of psychoanalysis. A psychoanalytic interpretation derives from these multiple contexts, which, following Lacan, I posit as signifying chains. Thus, in Lacan's theory of the subject, all identity, sameness, essence, and assurances are lost.[6]

All this is to a great extent, a consequence of Lacan's rejection of Saussure's linearity—another important issue to examine. Indeed, it is the standard view that thinking and speech occur as a succession of signifiers. As a consequence, the cure is conceived as an effect of the patient's free-flow of speech: "You just let him keep talking...." This is explicit in Colette Soler's work, whose notion of cure is similar to Freud's: it entails something like the lifting [*levantamiento*] of repression. In these accounts of the cure, a signifier is conceived as a word and in a linear manner, i.e., not as inserted in and bound to a signifying chain. The idea of a signifying loop, a link, also entails that, for Lacan, there is no signifier that is, taken as such, a master signifier. $S_1$ determines $S_2$ (anticipation) exactly as $S_2$ determines $S_1$ (retroaction): they are bound to each other in a circular entanglement.

The subject is thus divided between $S_1$ and $S_2$, which must be taken as a link chained to other links, which, as chains, are linked to other chains. Such a split has nothing to do with Freud's division of the psychic apparatus. The most important difference is that, for Lacan, the division is not internal to anyone. In fact, it is not even necessary that the patient utters anything through his mouth. Signifiers are not spoken words, but anything that can signify in a given, relevant discursive context.

It is on the basis of these ideas that Lacan develops an entirely new theory of the operations he calls "alienation" and "separation"—a theory that is completely lost in Lacanianism. Today, the prevailing version of psychoanalysis is oriented by the evolutionary and identitarian modern ideal according to which, in order to discover our own individual path, each of us must distinguish ourselves from our predecessors and our contemporaries. Romanticism, by promoting the ideal that each destiny must be individual, consolidated this movement. Further, an individual destiny is not easily achieved, for one is to differentiate oneself from all others. The "teenage crisis" demonstrates this eloquently: each young boy or girl is expected to express his or her individuality as distinct from his/her family and everyone in his/her milieu. But who is really able to come up with a genuinely personal, totally new idea? What most people think and communicate to others has been already maintained by others, including authors one has not read. This is why when a truly new idea emerges, its author makes history. These are the cases of Picasso and Dalí, Einstein and Newton, Lacan and Freud, etc.

Paradoxically, adolescents become rebellious and go through a crisis because of the obligation imposed on them by society. It has nothing to do with their testes and ovaries, as Freud thought (adolescence is seen by him as the end of latency and as the maturation of libido caused by gonadal pressure triggered by the individual's entering into puberty). Quite the contrary, it is the result of the obligation to be different and choose an identity at an early age imposed on them by society: "What will you study? What do you want to do with your life?" In practice, to be different is nothing more than imitation of someone else. There were times where even the figure of the hermit on the top of the mountain who never meets or talks to anyone became fashionable. Early Christianity, for instance, promoted the notion that depriving oneself of all pleasurable experiences and social relationships is an ideal to be achieved. Bosch's painting of the hermit saints shows it very well. Similarly, in Islam and Hinduism, one is expected to separate oneself from all others and remain in solitude for 30 days (the equivalent for us would be spending 30 minutes without the phone). "Isolate to find yourself"—this is a contradictory social and cultural demand. Let us recall that, after all, cloistered monks still exist.

### Alienation and Separation in Lacan's Theory of the Subject

The most common interpretation of alienation and separation in psychoanalysis coincides with a social ideal: we are born alienated from our parents and we are expected to separate ourselves from them (their demands, desires, norms, etc.) as we become adults. Lacanians call this "subjective constitution." Each of us is obligated to create and embrace his/her own difference.

Lacan's theory argues something else entirely, as shown particularly by his essay, "The Position of the Unconscious" and the first and second sessions of *Seminar XI*.

*Seminar XI* is the first seminar published during Lacan's lifetime. To my mind, however, his position is much better presented in his *Écrits'* essay.

Lacan's theory of alienation can be briefly stated as follows: The signifying loop, for Lacan, entails that neither $S_1$ nor $S_2$ stand alone, from which it follows that I am neither $S_1$ nor $S_2$ and, more radically, that "I am not." But what is it exactly that I am not? I am not an ego [*yo*], i.e., I am always an other to myself. Alienation means that each of us is an other: other to myself, but not other, different from the other/Other, as in the standard interpretation.

The subject that emerges as an effect of language and discourse is a subject characterized by two movements. The first one, alienation, was just described. As we are born into a signifying world, we have no identity proper, rather, we are born alienated from ourselves. A subject is a topic that will never be susceptible to definition, either by a word or by an idea. A swarm of terms of a signifying structure will have to be established for us to have a semblance of it. Consider the expression, "being Argentinean." What could this mean? One could reply, "Those who love Lionel Messi." But, obviously, not everyone does; some, in fact, despise him. Instead, it may be said, "Those who drink mate." But many do not, and there are non-Argentineans who drink it too, etc. In short, Lacan's conceptions entail that being itself is lost: every topic originated in the signifying dialectic will always be other to and other than itself.

Lacan argues that it is separation that can rescue us from alienation. This is the second movement, and has nothing to do with separation from our parents or our families. Quite the contrary, the movement entails a separation from the alienating effect of the articulation of signifiers. Lacan calls it, "the signifier's lethal effect:" the signifier kills the thing. Thus, the topic/issue/subject-matter to which we are linked and that we think we are is characterized by a lethal factor. The movement that yields the opposite effect is separation.

Lacan designates alienation's effect as "fading" (in English), i.e., the erasure of the subject. The subject appears between $S_1$ and $S_2$, but it appears erased, lacking being, consistency, identity, and essence. It appears and, synchronically, disappears. In each personal story, what rescues one from the signifier's lethal effect—the movement of separation—is one's falling into the place of the Other's object *a*, something that pertains to each person's particular story. Alienation happens because we live in a signifying world. In this sense, it may be said that it is intrinsic to *every* subject—it is its structure—as *every* subject is born into a signifying universe.

What rescues one from the signifier's lethal effect, from being-nothing, is being taken in a particular story as an other's object *a*. It is the opposite of what Lacanians hold. They claim that one is born alienated to the Other and one must separate oneself from it. What I am arguing is the exact reverse: we are born mortified, and what rescues us from this condition is being taken by the Other as an object *a*. Only at this point does the dialectic of the object start to operate. None of this is thematized by Freud or the Lacanians, as today virtually no one works with these ideas, which are to be found in a literal reading of Lacan. Thus, in each case, for each story, there is the possibility of occupying the place of the Other's object *a* (Lacan's formula of the *fantasme* is $ \lozenge $ a). Lacan argues that the condition of each story is the result of the way in which the Other's capture of the subject (topic/issue/subject-matter) takes place. In this movement, the subject, so construed, is taken as an object. Further, this capture is the reverse complement of the signifying alienation.

For Lacan, the time corresponding to the alienation/separation dialectic is also circular. One must conceive of a time that is synchronic but not simultaneous. For a language to emerge, one must also presuppose it, as Saussure presupposed, synchronically, all the terms of a language already existing. It is therefore inconceivable that there is first a mother, then a son, etc. In fact, what could "mother" even mean without "son"? Steven Pinker, the famous Harvard neuroscientist and author of *The Instinct of Language*, holds that language, and therefore the first speaker of a language, emerged out of a genetic mutation. On his resumé, he posted a CT scan of his brain and wrote underneath, "this is me." He is far the only one who has embraced this line of thought. In fact, there are still researchers examining Einstein's brain trying to find out how it worked and what there was inside. The reader may recall that Einstein was buried without his brain precisely because of the intention of examining it after his death.

Synchronic time entails that if we are to conceive a language, we must posit that all of its terms were there already. To speak of, say, a "mother," one must be able to refer to "son," but also to "grandmother;" otherwise, how would we refer to the mother of the mother? Obviously, the same applies to "father." This means that the whole of family institutions must already be there. The temporality of alienation and separation works in the same way. Due to their heavily Freudian filiation, most Lacanians work with an evolutionary theory: first, one is born alienated from his parents; then, once one is an adult, one must separate oneself from them. There is a progression to it. On the contrary, for Lacan, alienation and separation, as operations, entail an immixing with the other/Other.

The subject, as all signifiers, is and remains always blended with the Other/other. The same applies to $S_1$ and $S_2$, the condition of the subject and the object *a*, alienation and separation, analysand and analyst, etc. In the psychoanalytic tradition there is a very strong demand that the material is "what the patient says." They naively forget that what the patient says is what the analyst says that the patient said in a specific discursive context.

## On the Psychoanalytic Cure

On the basis of the previous discussion of Lacan's arguments, we can conclude that the cure is possible in psychoanalysis. The cure is what resolves what does not work or what causes suffering in the subject/topic. What is cured in an analysis is the conflict of that topic, the symptomatic dimension of the case, even when the analysand does not know anything about it. The cure is the case as seen from the subject's perspective, i.e., as it presents something that does not work in the discursive thread: a contradiction, aporia, or fallacy. Thus, we have an answer to the question about the end of an analysis and the orientation of the cure. An analysis does not change people; it resolves what does not work well in the material, understood in a structural manner (one can think of a case as a defective machine). What can be cured is the symptom of the topic, not the character's traits. Psychoanalysis does not make people better.

We need, therefore, to distinguish between different concepts: "analysand," "analyst," and "subject." Keep in mind what was discussed earlier: it may be that the patient schedules a consultation with the analyst because he thinks he is "depressed" as a consequence of losing his "job," but over the course of a session it is found out that the real issue is that his wife will be "leaving" him for not having and not being able to make money. It could even be the case that it becomes about something else, say, that his wife will leave him because once his father-in-law, "the father of his wife," lost his job and fell into a serious depression, as a consequence of which the wife told the patient, "I don't want a depressing person at home," which could, in turn, be articulated to the story of the patient's parents, etc. In sum, through the analysis of the subject by both analyst and analysand, an immixing chain of alterity [*otredad*] is constituted, which is the topic, the issue of an analysis. This is why Lacan claims that there is a "new subject" only if an analysis reaches a successful end, something he thematizes under the rubric of the analytic act. Only from this perspective can one understand the notion of a new subject, as this is not at all a new person. It is the problem in the topic that changes, not the subject as an individual.

Accordingly, Lacan introduces a new account of the symptom: *Symptôme,* a neologism coined from the ancient French. For Lacan, *symptôme* admits a topological correlate, for when he manages to create the figures of the analyst and the analysand. The pass is theoretically operative with the Borromean knot in such a way that it has a specific logical expression as the fourth ring of a Brunnian link. Inherent to the latter is the fact that if one ring is removed, the rest are freed, too. As a rule, Lacanians do not work with the idea of an immixing of alterity. As a consequence, they develop a theory based on the notion of responsibility, which, in turn, is attributed to someone, an individual. In APOLa we do work with the idea of an immixing of alterity, as we work within a scientifically-oriented program that makes of such a notion one of its premises. The subject is thus conceived as something to be understood and established always in an immixing of alterity (Other/other). The *symptôme* as a knotting is what is cut in an analysis when its end is attained. Overall, it is a term that most Freudo-Lacanians have forgotten, as for Freud there is no such a thing as an immixing of alterity. This is why, for him, one is responsible for the content of one's dreams. Because dreams are ours, the expression of our desires and our drives, who else could be responsible for them but us? For Freud, lived experiences and their representations are individual (they belong to an individual internally divided); the psychic apparatus is within the person, it is internal to the person. It is clear, then, that Freud defends a theoretical and practical model that is heavily individualistic, the exact opposite of Lacan's.

## Notes

1 This is an edited version of a talk given at the Ramos Mejía Hospital in Buenos Aires, Argentina, on August 1, 2019.
2 It should be noted that, primarily because of the global expansion of technology, almost all cultures are fundamentally permeated by the concepts, ways of living, life-styles, etc., that constitute what is commonly called "the West."
3 On this topic, the reader may consult Jean-Luc Nancy's "Un Sujet," in Weil, Dominique (ed.), Homme et sujet: la subjectivité en question dans les sciences humaines (Paris: Editions L'Harmattan, 1993), pp. 47–115. Nancy studied Lacan very carefully; the book is a series of talks given by Nancy to Lacanian psychoanalysts. Lacan discussed the issue in the 24th session of his *Seminar II*, which he entitled "A-M-A-S," the extremes of the Z scheme. "Amas" means "nebulae" in French. He also discussed the issue in "Position of the Unconscious and the Dialectics of the Freudian Unconscious" (in the *Écrits*) and the Baltimore presentation, "Structure as the Inmixing of Otherness as a Prerequisite to Any Subject Whatsoever."
4 The Spanish term literally means "burial," "entombment," and captures some of the semantic aspects of the term "Untergang" in the title of Freud's 1924 essay, "*Untergang des Oedipuscomplexes*." Stratchey's translation is "dissolution," which, as shown by what follows in Eidelsztein's text, is misleading [Translator's note; hereafter, "TN"].
5 See his *The Society of Individuals* (New York & London: Continuum, 1991). This book includes an unbeatable chapter on adolescence. Notice the paradox entailed in the title.
6 These claims oppose J.-A. Miller's—*not Lacan's*—theory of the unitary trait, as Miller develops a psychoanalysis founded on the idea that there is a primary trace of the drive's jouissance in the anatomical, real body, one that does *not* work as Lacan's signifier, but as Freud's mnemic trace.

# Chapter 3

# The Origin of the Subject in Psychoanalysis. On the Big Bang of Language and Discourse

## The Problem of the Origin of the Subject in Freud and Lacan

The problem of origin is a topic seldom raised and examined in theoretical and clinical discussions among psychoanalysts, particularly in connection with the origin of the subject. To my mind, this is one of the most difficult and important issues in psychoanalysis.

Sigmund Freud and Jacques Lacan developed full-fledged theories about it. Freud's is evolutionist in nature; Lacan's is creationist. Such difference persists both at the level of the analysis of particular cases as well as of society as a whole.

The evolutionist approach starts off by positing a beginning from something substantial, tangible, something that evolves and develops until maturity is reached (at the level of the particular being, the latter entails the constitution of a biological entity, at least a unicellular one; at the level of society, the primal horde). On the contrary, the creationist one starts off by positing nothingness (ex nihilo creation), rejecting thereby the notions of evolution and maturity.

As Freud's position is well known, it will not be presented through recourse to quotations and arguments. Besides, it coincides with our common sense and the view defended by many scientists in other disciplines, such as biology, neurology, and genetics. On the contrary, Lacan's position is ignored and rejected even by his disciples and followers. This is the view, then, that must be recuperated.

As attested to by the following claims, Lacan, from the beginning to the end of his teaching, defended the creationist argument:

| | | |
|---|---|---|
| The symbol... | ...is already operative from the beginning. | Seminar II, 16th class |
| The Other... | ...is already in its locus in the system of the world. | Seminar III, sixth class |
| Signification... | ...is always at stake in what pertains to the subject. | Seminar III, 15th class |

DOI: 10.4324/9781003485339-5

| The Other... | ...is always in ourselves. | Seminar III, fifteenth class |
|---|---|---|
| The Other... | ...is already instated in that spot [that of natural desire]. | Seminar VIII, fifteenth class |
| The Other... | ...precedes any subjective revelation. | Seminar XI, tenth class |
| The Other... | ...is already present each time that the unconscious opens up. | Seminar XI, tenth class |
| Language... | ...is already efficaciously present in every manifestation of the unary trait. | Seminar XVII, eleventh class |
| One can only speak of jouissance... | ...as something linked to the very origin of the mise-en-scène of the signifier. | Seminar XVIII, first class |
| The society of signifiers... | ...is a necessary condition for the emergence and the refusal of the master signifier ($S_1$). | Seminar XVIII, first class |

Lacan's proposal, systematically defended throughout his work, was an absolute novelty in psychoanalysis. However, as evidenced by the fact that barely any psychoanalysts hold it today, the proposal is now almost extinct.

Let us first examine its consequences. From the thesis that both A (i.e., the locus of the treasure and battery of the signifiers, of truth and logic, posited by Lacan as Ⱥ due to its intrinsic lack) and the Other[1] (i.e., its historical embodiment) are always already in their locus, two conclusions may be drawn:

1  As indicated by the term "battery," A and the Other are complete. This is the case even though their lack is ineliminable and the fact that they entail a series of impossibilities (hence the "treasure" of signifiers).
2  No one, neither a person nor a group, could have produced them.

Lacan posits two operations to account for the subject's causation: alienation and separation. These operations have been widely mentioned among his followers; however, they tend to ignore that in Lacan's theoretical model, the notions of **subject** and **cause** are endowed with very specific meanings. If one is to examine the origin of the subject rigorously, it is imperative to study them in detail.

Lacan's concept of subject—"the Lacanian subject"[2]—does not coincide with the (biological) individual, the (social and historical) person, the (legal and political) citizen, or the member (of a group). Neither does the analysand, in Lacan's teaching, coincide with the subject. Further, the analysand is conceived as a *parlêtre*,[3] a neologism coined by Lacan to reject the *being* in "human being." Thus, "parlêtre" (1) indicates that being is created in and through speaking, (2) refers to *a* being in its particular condition, not to a common feature of a plurality of beings, and (3) introduces the polyphony—a plurality of voices—of the otherness' *inmixing* (i.e., a mixing in which the composing elements can no longer be distinguished), rejecting thereby the individualistic interpretation of "human being" as *a*-speaking-*being*.

**Cause** does not refer to what preceded a fact or to a necessary relation between facts. Aware of the standard meaning of the term, Lacan claims, as do many other authors, that it is always a limping cause.[4] Thus, "subject" and "cause" are resignified and defined reciprocally as follows:

1 Language causes the subject:
   The weight we attribute to language as the cause of the subject....[5]
2 If language causes the subject, then it is impossible that the subject is the cause of itself:
   The effect of language is the cause introduced into the subject. Through this effect, the subject is not the cause of itself; it bears within itself the worm of the cause that splits it.[6]
3 Lacan is obliged to claim that it is not so much language in general, but the signifying [*significante*] order in its particularity that which must be placed as the cause of the subject:
   Because its cause is the signifier, without which there would be no subject in the real.[7]
4 The signifier is not a term of any particular language (as in linguistics):
   A subject intervenes only inasmuch as there are, in this world, signifiers that mean nothing and must be deciphered.[8]
5 The subject will then be defined through Lacan's canonical formula: "the subject is what represents a signifier for another signifier:"
   But this subject is what the signifier represents, and the latter cannot represent anything except for another signifier.[9]
6 Lastly, for Lacan, the cause consists in adopting the ethical and theoretical stance of a rationality that claims that the subject is a signifier's effect:
   For the cause is not, as is said of being as well, a lure of forms of discourse—otherwise it would have already been dispelled. It perpetuates the reason that subordinates the subject to the signifier's effect.[10]

If the signifying order is the cause of the subject and the latter is not the biological individual affected by language, its subject could never have been produced with substantial raw materials, such as the biological body of evolutionary theory. On the contrary, the subject is *created* (creationist theory), i.e., it comes to exist out of **nothingness**. The latter can be thought of as (a) the fact that a signifier as such does not mean anything,[11] (b) the empty interval among signifiers,[12] and (c) the holes in the Borromean knot [*cadena*] originated by the signifying loop [*bucle*].

These notions entail a radical change in the conceptualization of time and space in the psychoanalytic clinic.

Time will now be reversible, which implies that:

1  time is circular;
2  the present is lost;
3  the future logically precedes over the past.

These properties of time are designated by Lacan as "future perfect tense" [*future antérieur*][13] or what I prefer to call, "past future without present:"

> [This closing also] demonstrates the core of a reversion time, quite necessarily introduced to explain the efficiency of discourse....

and

> [Alienation and separation] are sorted out in a circular relation.[14]

None of this was conceived in this manner by Freud. Even if his conception of the unconscious' temporality entails the notion of *nachträglichkeit*,[15] Lacan was the first psychoanalyst to emphasize it, transforming it into his *après-coup*.[16] one should not forget that Freud utilizes the notion to account for two phenomena:

1  The reinterpretation of infantile trauma during the second wave of genital maturation. The notion acquires, thus, a sexual connotation.
2  The infantile lived-experiences [*vivencias*] that have a retroactive effect.

However, for Freud, trauma and infantile lived-experiences are events that took place in the past, and their resignification or delayed manifestation will occur in the future. Both lived experience and trauma, operating as real references, take place in the present.

Let us keep in mind that the account of time in the modern theories of the universe is absolutely different from Freud's and also from the everyday beliefs of the majority of people. Further, physics works under the presupposition (one that has strong empirical support) that the researcher's intervention modifies the results of research (a basic principle of quantum mechanics) and, further, alters the past or, more rigorously, the pasts of what is being investigated.[17]

I propose that the same applies to the practice of psychoanalysis.

Indeed, one of the effects looked after in the course of a psychoanalytic treatment is the institution of different pasts. Such an effect can be seen as a genuine creation of these pasts and, therefore, as being much more than the mere resignification of indelible and permanent historical events, such as Freud's "mnemic traces." I will later return to this issue.

In the Freudian model, the constitution of the psychic apparatus presupposes (i) the taking-place of a real phenomenon, (ii) its subsequent inscription as a trace, and (iii) its articulation in words. In contrast, through his concepts of signifier and subject, Lacan posits that, at the level of the subject, there is nothing prior to the

signifying order and the Other, enabling thereby the existence of "signifying phenomena," which amounts to the erasure of all real references. Such phenomena
take place in a time that is different from linear time.

For Lacan, space is mathematical in nature: it is the space of a topological surface characterized as a bi-dimensional combinatory of points. In his view, the function of the hole is crucial. He writes,

> The structure of what closes [*se ferme*] is, indeed, inscribed in a geometry
> in which space is reduced to a combinatory: it is what is called an "edge" in
> topology.[18]

According to Freud's conception of space, particularly as developed in the so-called
"second topography" (the one that psychoanalysts tend to embrace the most), the
psychic apparatus is posited as a tri-dimensional egg and thought of as internal to
the natural body. For Freud, what is important in the erogenous zones is the skin's
outskirts—but only because of the high nerve-sensitivity of its outer parts. In the
Lacanian model, the subject is signifying and the space that corresponds to it is
therefore a bi-dimensional one. Indeed, in the signifying universe there are only two
dimensions: the metaphorical (substitution) and the metonymical (connection). The
former can be represented as a "vertical" axis and the latter as a "horizontal" one. By
reference to the typical way of writing in the Western, modern languages—horizontal
and proceeding from left to right—the distinction can be depicted as follows:

Metaphor
(vertical)

Metonymy
(horizontal)

It is also possible to tabulate the differences between Freud and Lacan in their
conceptualization of time as shown in the following scheme:

| Sigmund Freud | Jacques Lacan |
| --- | --- |
| Infantile trauma → Sexual maturation (past: zero to five years-old) (future: 10–12-years-old) | 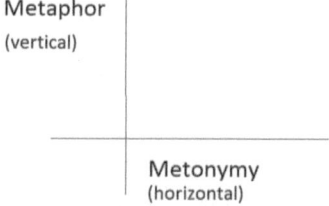 The second signifier is the cause of the first one (and vice versa); no signifier is, in itself, the past or the future of the other. |
| Linear time (arrow of time) | Circular time |

Such differences, actively ignored among Lacanian authors, are made even more explicit when Lacan proposes a critical revision of the Freudian stages: oral, anal, phallic, etc.

| Sigmund Freud | Jacques Lacan |
|---|---|
| oral → anal → phallic → genital | 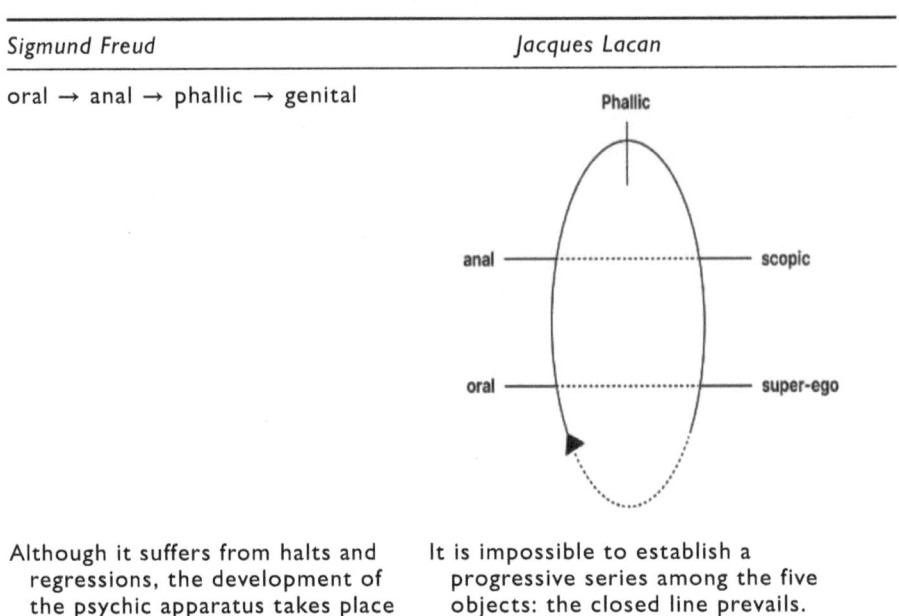 |
| Although it suffers from halts and regressions, the development of the psychic apparatus takes place along a linear chronological axis, from a primitive origin to the mature stages. | It is impossible to establish a progressive series among the five objects: the closed line prevails. |

One may also find Lacan's conception of circular time operating in his elaboration of **alienation** and **separation**, to which I have already briefly referred. Lacan's disciples divulged these notions, interpreting them as terms referring to an evolutionary process: first, we are born alienated to the Other and then we must separate ourselves from it to become "ourselves." Lacan, quite remarkably, does the exact opposite:

> It is thus not the fact that this operation begins in the Other that leads me to call it "alienation."[19]

Thus, **alienation** is the advent of the subject as it is split between two signifiers and localized in the interval between them, which prevents the subject from being one or the other. It is an operation that establishes that one cannot be oneself, something that Lacan designates as lack of being, *manque à être*, as well as the signifier's lethal factor.[20]

**Separation** consists in the articulation of the subject's lack of being with the lack that manifests itself in the intervals in the Other's signifying chain. As a consequence, the subject may find its locus in these other intervals, which, in turn, opens up the possibility that it becomes the object of the Other's desire. In short, contrary to the standard view in psychoanalytic circles, it is the Other that rescues the subject.[21]

As there cannot be alienation without the conditions imposed by the existence of the signifying pair that necessarily introduces the Other, it is evident that the time of the two operations is circular.[22]

Lacan puts it as follows:
Therein lies the twist whereby separation represents the return of alienation.[23]
As for the spatial hole, Lacan and Freud's views also differ:

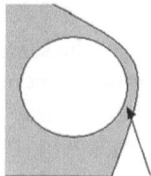 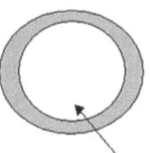

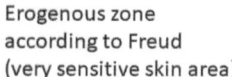

Erogenous zone
according to Freud
(very sensitive skin area)

Erogenous zone
according to Lacan
(hole)

For Freud, the spatial hole is the strongly innervated skin around the bodily orifices. Lacan, on the contrary, speaks of the hole's function,[24] which sets up the signifying loop in the anatomical body.

In Lacan's last seminars, it is the hole, topologically defined, that, even more accurately than the signifying interval, creates and accommodates the nothingness of the ex nihilo creation in the Borromean knot. Such a hole is also the place of creation and that of the engulfing whirl[25,26] of material substances.[27] The hole functions as the locus where $, A, and the object *a* exist—the place where, for the *parlêtre*, the material function of the tri-dimensional substances dissolves. Once the usage of the Borromean knot is mobilized, the modalities of *jouissance*, j(A) and j(φ), will also be thought of by Lacan as residing in the holes, which means they cannot be assumed to be the *jouissance* of a bodily substance.

A few additional clarifications on the notion of time are in order. From his seminar on transference, Lacan argues (in a way entirely consistent with the above considerations) that if one is to account for the origin of natural languages [*lenguas*] it is necessary to hold that all its elements emerged not simultaneously, but synchronically.

To my mind, Lacan was never more explicit about it than in this passage:

Language is inaugural in a different sense. It has to do with this dimension that language institutes as synchrony, which is a completely different thing than simultaneity.[28]

"Simultaneous" refers to two events happening at the same chronological moment. "Synchronic" is an abstraction that accounts for the origin of all natural languages or, more rigorously (putting it in terms of Lacan's model), all signifying sets. Further, it indicates that the structure as a whole is already there from the beginning, including what it lacks and what is impossible in it. Let us notice that such time does not admit of any periodization or chronology (i.e., it does not coincide with the time of clocks and calendars).

Lacan rejects the possibility that there is a first signifier to which other signifiers are added in temporal succession. If we return to the chart presented on pp. 24, the quotations from *Seminars XVII* and *XVIII* clearly show that Lacan holds that the society of signifiers is a necessary condition for the emergence [*nacimiento*] and disavowal [*rechazo*] of $S_1$, language for the unitary trait, and the signifying interplay for *jouissance*.

In *Writing and Difference*, Jacques Derrida proposes the same temporal logic for his notion of structure, characterized by him as having no center, origin, or end.[29] Further, he makes clear, in agreement with Lacan, that the structure must be posited as "always being there." This is not, however, how we tend to think about it, for we are more used to a reasoning along these lines:

> Where did this linguistic-alphabetical Tower of Babel come from, anyway? How does a particular alphabet arise? At some primal point, at the very beginning, it had to start with a single sign, a single character. Someone made a mark in order to remember something. Or to communicate something to someone else. Or to cast a spell on an object or a territory.
>
> But why do different people describe the same object with so many completely different notations? All over the world a man, a mountain, or a tree look much alike, and yet in each alphabet different symbols, images, or letters correspond to them. Why is it that the very first individual who wanted to describe a flower made a vertical line in one culture, a circle in another culture, and in a third decided on two lines and a cone?[30]

Ryszard Kapuściński defends a widespread order [*legalidad*] of thinking that goes against Lacan's. In the quotation above one immediately notices that the logic of the "first sign" requires one to posit a "first being."

Justifying Lacan's position requires a highly meticulous and careful argumentation. It is also necessary to clarify what may appear as a contradiction in his conceptualization of time, namely, that he claims both its circularity and its absolute beginning.

Let us delve into the arguments further.

For Lacan, time must be conceived as circular—in correspondence to the logic of the future anterior—for all discursive experience, understood as a social link in which the participants are *parlêtres*. Now, when it comes to the origin of language and the subject, one must accept a non-dateable, absolute, synchronic beginning. All this implies the notion of an "always already there."

I would like now to propose that we abandon those old, already surpassed scientific theories, still utilized (even inadvertently) by most psychoanalysts, and embrace a contemporary scientific model, one required to account for the absolute beginning of language, the Other, and the subject. This is, to my mind, an indispensable epistemological maneuver aimed to resolve contradictions internal to psychoanalysis.

Based on my own research, my conviction is that the whole of Lacan's theoretical developments establishes that to account for the subject (and its functions, sensations, affects, needs, etc.), one must posit the preexistence of the signifying order and the Other as its causal reason. From this it follows that everything that seems to come from the *parlêtre's* biological body is in fact *created*. As such, it is absolutely different from any animal or biological phenomenon.

A subject, contrary to a person, a citizen, an individual, or a member of a group [*un socio*], is not a member of any animal species. Thus, the position I am defending rejects any identification between Lacan's subject and a "speaking animal" (in the many ways in which one can account for the latter).[31] If this were not the case, one should admit that what occurs to certain animals could also occur to the subject, as in the case of domesticated dogs, whose instincts (primal and internal), when subjected to conditioning (secondary and external), are significantly modified. In the theoretical model I defend, both drive [*pulsión*] and *jouissance* are the concepts aiming to prevent that the logic of conditioning from being applied to the subject of psychoanalytic practice.

From the fact that human life is always lived in a particular culture and society it is usually concluded that although both men and women are born endowed with natural drives, these are conditioned by society and culture. As a result, there is left a residue of "discontent"—hence Freud's well-known "civilization and its discontents." In this view, the sole difference between humans and animals—and it is conceived as a difference only of degree—lies in the fact that human conditioning is at most much more complex than the conditioning of animals. I find it necessary to argue against this stance.

Lacan's position is as clear as it is decisive: there is no pre-discursive reality.[32] This means that the reality of the *parlêtre* is preceded by discourse, which necessarily entails that the articulation of signifiers and other *parlêtres* has already been operative. To summarize, there is always the primacy of the Other and the signifying order.

How to solve this new, apparent contradiction? What should one consider to have come first at the level of the subject: the animal-biological body or the signifying register in the context of discourse? With Lacan, I defend the latter view, because it is the only view that allows a robust justification of the nature of the analyst's function.

## The Question of the Origin from a Philosophical Perspective

Let us now return to the question of origin, this time from a philosophical perspective. Freud, following Goethe, posits that in the beginning there was the deed.[33]

On the contrary, for Lacan, following St. John's Gospel, in the beginning there was the word.[34]

How is it possible that there are signifiers—all of them existing synchronically—and the locus of the Other, with all its lack and impossibility, *before* there are human beings capable of both enunciating and understanding them?

For the vast majority of (or possibly all) Lacanian psychoanalysts, this opposition between a biological origin of the subject and an origin in language and discourse is understood as the opposition between *jouissance* (which they believe to be original and stemming from living substance) and the signifiers bound up with the Other, which, for them, appear at a second stage. Given that Lacan argues in the exact opposite direction, such a view is nothing but striking.

Indeed, for Lacan, what there is from the beginning is the signifying order and the Other and their effects: subject, truth, *jouissance*, lack, object *a*, drives, etc. In opposition, his disciples claim that what exists first is a living substance with its specific biological modalities of *jouissance*, which they posit as being singular.[35] Later, the signifier will attempt to grasp this *jouissance* in its web, achieving only partial victories. Lacan posits that *jouissance* exists because of the preexistence of the signifying order and the Other, precisely as an effect of their existence.

In "Subversion of the Subject and the Dialectic of Desire in the Freudian Unconscious," Lacan presents his conception of *jouissance*, new to psychoanalysis, in its most detailed form. Referring to $\sqrt{-1}$, he writes,

> This is what the subject is missing in thinking he is exhaustively accounted for by his cogito—he is missing what is unthinkable about him. But where does this being, who appears in some way missing from the sea of proper names, come from?
>
> We cannot ask this question of the subject qua *I* [*Je*]. He is missing everything he needs in order to know the answer, since if this subject, *I*, was dead [*moi J'étais mort*], he would not know it, as I said earlier. Thus, he does not know I am alive. How, therefore, will *I* prove it to myself?
>
> For I can, at most, prove to the Other that he exists, not, of course, with the proofs of the existence of God with which the centuries have killed him, but by loving him, a solution introduced by the Christian kerygma.
>
> It is, in any case, too precarious a solution for us to even think of using it to circumvent our problem, namely: What am *I* [*Je*]?
>
> *I* am in the place from which "the universe is a flaw in the purity of Non-Being" is vociferated.
>
> And not without reason for, by protecting itself, this place makes Being itself languish. This place is called *Jouissance*, and it is *Jouissance* whose absence would render the universe vain.[36]

In this remarkable passage, one among many, it is very clearly asserted that *jouissance* operates as that which responds to the question, "What am I?," i.e., as something that pertains to the problems of being and the I as they appear only to *parlêtres* that exist in the modality of a "lack of being" in specific historical, social, and cultural contexts. Lacan shows that *jouissance* responds to these problems as $\sqrt{-1}$ responds to the problem of being as it is raised in the universe of so-called "natural" numbers. The concept of *jouissance* indicates that the latter appears in the place from which it was vociferated that the universe is a flaw of plenitude—even the lack's. If one agrees with Lacan's thesis, how is it possible to claim that *jouissance* comes from living substance, when it is clearly required that "the universe is a flaw in the purity of Non-Being" is previously vociferated?

The problem raised by $\sqrt{-1}$ in the context of a discussion of the notions of subject and *jouissance* also appears when one examines the issue of the origin of numbers. In relation to natural numbers, the problem appears as follows: it is not the case that 1 emerged before 2, 2 before 3, and so on and so forth. On the contrary, all the elements of the structure came to be all together, not one by one. Along the same lines, then, the notion that $S_1$ came to be before $S_2$ must be rejected. Naturally, the same applies to the subscripts of these signifiers. Hans Reichenbach, the main representative of what is known as "scientific philosophy," puts it as follows:

> Here we meet with a development which manifests the relative independence of a mathematical formalism; the mathematical symbols have a life of their own, so to speak, and lead to the correct result even before the symbol-user understands their ultimate meaning.[37]

Let us return to our issue: Can there be signifiers and the Other before a flesh—and by the latter I mean our genes and neurons—capable of producing and hosting them? What kind of substance would they require? These questions are guided by the ongoing Western prejudice—not at all a modern one[38]—that affirms that for there to be thinking, doubt, etc., there must exist, prior in time, an individual I anchored in a biological body. Although not well-known, this is a long debate of at least eight centuries. It can be summarized as follows: Is it necessary to posit a tri-dimensional substance as the host of thought?

For Lacan, as for St. Augustin, Averroes, G.C. Lichtenberg, F.W.J. Schelling, F. Nietzsche, C. Lévi-Strauss, A. Rimbaud, P. Ricoeur, A. de Libera, M. Angenot, among others, "*Es denkt in mir*,"[39] "It thinks in me." A psychoanalytic clinic built around this thesis is very different from one articulated around its rejection, for instance, in the name of any figure of subjective responsibility or involvement.[40]

For Freud there must always be someone doing the thinking and psychoanalysis can only exist as long as individual, moral responsibility for one's unconscious thoughts is recognized.[41] Freud thinks that one is ultimately responsible for what one thinks and does. On the contrary, Lacan argues that "It *(ça)* thinks alone," a claim that is at the heart of his account of the unconscious:

> One therefore does not speak to the subject. It speaks of him…[42]

A consequence of positing that "It thinks alone…" is that plagiarism becomes logically impossible:[43] no one has ever owned any thought. This is why Lacan explicitly claims that intellectual property does not exist; this notion is for him mere prejudice.[44] Thoughts are thought by "It" *(ça)*, a term that indicates that Freud's *Id* has been transformed into a non-individual instance.

In his remarkable, indispensable research on the archeology of the subject, A. de Libera labels Freud's position, "attributivism." This is a view that posits the subject as a responsible or, to put it in more modern terms, as an imputable subject.[45]

Like the rest of the psychoanalytic community, the Lacanian movement today, both in its theoretical as well as its clinical components, revolves around the notion of subjective responsibility. This is the exact opposite of the view defended by Lacan:

> This is even what Freud discovered precisely around 1920, and this is, in a way, the retrogressive point of his discovery. His discovery was to have spelt out the unconscious and I defy anyone to say that this could be anything other than the remark that there is a perfectly articulated knowledge for which, properly speaking, no subject is responsible.[46]

We now arrive at the main thesis of this essay.

## The Origin of the Subject and the Big Bang Theory

It is worth insisting that when defending their ideas, psychoanalysts make use of outdated scientific models that have already been substituted by others. However, most of them seem to remain unaware of this. I propose that psychoanalytic theory could benefit from making use of the logic of one of the main theories in modern cosmological physics: the big bang theory.[47] As I will show, this theory serves as an instrument to help us reach a rational solution for the alleged contradictions of an account of the subject that posits it as having been created ex nihilo.

The big bang theory, widely accepted in the scientific world for more than half a century, holds that the universe, including all of its matter and space-time, had an absolute beginning 13.5 billion years ago. It is not necessary for the theory to posit the inexistence of what was before the big bang; it logically suffices that the theory claims that, if there is such a thing, it has no causal power. Stephen Hawking explains it as follows:

> All of the Friedmann solutions have the feature that at some time in the past (between ten and twenty thousand million years ago) the distance between neighboring galaxies must have been zero. At that time, which we call the big bang, the density of the universe and the curvature of space-time would have been infinite. Because mathematics cannot really handle infinite numbers, this means that the general theory of relativity (on which Friedmann's solutions are based) predicts that there is a point in the universe where the theory itself breaks down. Such a point is an example of what mathematicians call a singularity. In fact, all our theories of science are formulated on the assumption that space-time is smooth and nearly flat, so they break down at the big bang singularity, where

the curvature of space-time is infinite. This means that even if there were events before the big bang, one could not use them to determine what would happen afterward, because predictability would break down at the big bang.

Correspondingly, if, as is the case, we know only what has happened since the big bang, we could not determine what happened beforehand. As far as we are concerned, events before the big bang can have no consequences, so they should not form part of a scientific model of the universe. We should therefore cut them out of the model and say that time had a beginning at the big bang.[48]

Those who are not familiar with this theory (otherwise already considered a "classic theory") may be surprised to read that time is thought to have started with the big bang. But there is more. Space (physical space) also started with the beginning of time. In fact, in these models, including relativity theory, space-time is one sole object, a continuum, described and conceived by modern physics only and exclusively through mathematical language. We should bear in mind that common sense is still Aristotelian-Ptolemaic or, at best, for a cultivated person, Cartesian-Newtonian. Due to the ignorance in regards to scientific developments (even when, like the big bang theory, some of them are already a century old), it may also come as a surprise to many that, for modern physics, light is also an object.

More recent studies (2009) show that:

...it is difficult, if not impossible, for us to see directly back before the big bang....[49]

In his arguments, Martin Bojowald, a prominent physicist working on problems regarding the origin of the universe, makes use of the notion of **forgetfulness**:

...the universe, as it were, forgets which precise value such a property had taken before the big bang.[50]

This forgetting of everything that preceded the origin of the universe is designated by him as "cosmic forgetfulness."[51] Bojowald is obligated to acknowledge that despite recent attempts (including his own), attaining knowledge of the universe before the big bang is a utopian dream:

A direct image of the big bang itself, or even of the previous universe, remains a fantasy....[52]

In Stephen Hawking and Leonard Mlodinow's "The Grand Design," one finds the same argument about the effects of what existed before the big bang:

It is not yet clear whether a model in which time continued back beyond the big bang would be better at explaining present observations because it seems the laws of the evolution of the universe may break down at the big bang. If they do, it would make no sense to create a model that encompasses time before the big bang, because what existed then would have no observable consequences for the present, and so we might as well stick with the idea that the big bang was the creation of the world.[53]

In one of the best popular-science texts on the big bang theory, Alejandro Gangui also refers to this impossibility,only that this time the physical phenomena that occurred in the early instants after the big bang fall under its effects. As this point it should not come as a surprise that he, too, bases his argument on the notion of forgetfulness:

> But the continuous interactions prior to the recombination are responsible for the photons' "forgetfulness" of the information that they carried within themselves. This is why a direct access (at least through electromagnetic radiation) to the physical phenomena prior to that moment in time will always be veiled for us. The recombination is then like a "barrier" one cannot go around when attempting to look back into the "origin" of the expansion of the universe.[54]

This is, therefore, a widely, almost universally accepted theory among physicists and cosmologists. It includes those working within the relativistic and quantum-mechanistic perspectives as well as those doing research within more recent paradigms. Again, the theory claims that there was an absolute beginning that forgets what was before it (because, as explained, it is impossible to know) and, further, that after the beginning, what came before lacks the power to affect what exists from that point forward.

## The Logic of Time and Cause as Seen from the Perspective of the Big Bang Theory

The guiding thread of this book consists in making clear that applying the notion of absolute time, as conceived by common sense, Newtonian physics, and evolutionary logic, to the subject, as conceptualized in Lacan's teaching, ends up in a contradiction. Instead, I propose that psychoanalysis make use of the logic of time and cause as we find it in the big bang theory. This is the logic required by the concepts of subject and Other that should guide all psychoanalytic practice that proclaims itself oriented around Lacan's teaching.

There are at least two physical models of reality and the real: the one proposed by Newtonian physics and that of relativity theory, quantum mechanics, and the physics of strings and loops. The former can be seen as valid when interpreted as a limit case of the theoretical basis of the latter. Newtonian physics only works adequately for, say, the displacement of animal bodies in the three-dimensional space on Earth—it does not apply to interstellar or subatomic spaces.

Acknowledging the hegemony of the biological paradigm in the reflection on the subject, my contention is that everything that belongs to the domain of culture, society, language, history, etc., and, in particular, to the psychoanalytic subject, cannot be thought of on the basis of Newtonian physics—a model that operates with tri-dimensional, substantial particles like billiard balls invested with energy and moving around in eternal time and space.

It is imperative that we abandon such a model and welcome, in psychoanalysis, the kind of logic operative in the physical theories produced in the early twentieth century. These theories built the big bang model, as well as the concepts of field and waves in constant interweaving. Only this way could one speak, with Lacan, of *The Function and the Field of Speech and Language in Psychoanalysis*[55] and related sciences.

The big bang theory advances the idea that the whole universe emerges out of a single point that lacks any volume and has infinite energy: space, time, the matter that constitutes macroscopic material objects (including human bodies), etc., all comes out of it.

I propose that the logic utilized by modern science in the big bang theory to account for the origin of the universe is the most suitable for understanding the origin and the structure of the subject in Lacan's theory and in psychoanalytic practice. There are two reasons for this:

1  It is a way of making Lacan's arguments on the "being already there" of language and the Other more coherent. When it comes to the specific phenomena of psychoanalytic clinic, then, the biological body will have to be "forgotten."
2  It grounds the notion that no human being or group created language or the unconscious. Similarly, one should not posit the existence of a subject before the unconscious, or that the latter is a consequence of a series of experiences, pleasurable or otherwise, lived by someone. The unconscious, as the Other's discourse and structured as a language, is and has always been already there, after an absolute beginning that cannot be dated. One is not obligated to deny the "prior" existence of the biological body, but there is, nonetheless, an *absolute discontinuity*, a radical forgetfulness of the biological order in order to enter into the discursive one.

Although I have not found any evidence that Lacan explicitly articulated his theory with the big bang model,[56] his theory requires a conception of time according to the temporal and causal logic of the big bang theory as the most modern scientific model of the universe. We should thrive for a psychoanalysis that, like Lacan's teaching, remains always intimately and constantly related to the most subversive and surprising developments in quantum and relativistic physics.[57]

To sum up, I propose a consideration of Lacan's concept of the subject along the same logic used by the physicists of our time. The emergence of the signifier, the battery, and the Other operates as a big bang. This means that for the subject and all its effects in psychoanalytic practice and the sciences of culture and society, the biological, animal order is "forgotten"—something I call, "**lack of biological memory**." The emergence of language and the Other entails an absolute discontinuity with what was before it, which applies in particular to the loss of the biological body, forgotten in its natural condition. This is so in each particular case as well as in every dimension of society and culture.

Both the biological body of the newly born baby as well as the body of the anthropoid group before the emergence of language must be considered as entirely lacking their causal power:

> ...what 'there was' [the entity {*el ser*}] disappears, as it is no longer anything but a signifier".[58]

From the existence of language and the Other, the anatomical body too becomes a signifier. This was Freud's discovery in relation to the hysterical symptom. However, Freud was unable to theorize it because he could not get rid of the Newtonian and biologistic models, both of them major components of the paradigm that was becoming predominant in the West.[59]

Thus, what I am rejecting is not only the notion that there was a first term to which, at a second stage, another term was added:[60] what I am arguing is that once the synchronic "big explosion" of the emergence of language occurred, everything that happened and existed before it was forgotten. The alleged first term, sign, or signal, of the otherwise so convincing evolutionary theory of language, cannot have a place in any language, for the elements of the latter (as it is also the case with the elements of a set in the mathematical theory of sets) exist only as elements of a structure and as such they are synchronically different from all others, i.e., all together or not at all. Of course, there are signs in the animal world, but they are not signifiers. If a sign is operative for the *parlêtre*, it is because it is already a signifier. When elements are integrated into a language, as when they disappear (as it constantly happens), they are all modified in a covariant manner.

Let us return to Kapuściński's text. It will be useful to clarify how the idea of a big bang of language and discourse is necessary to respond to the genuinely important questions:

> All right, then—let's say, thirty to fifty individuals. Such is the nucleus of a tribe. But why does such a nucleus necessarily come to need its own language?[61] How could the human mind even invent such an astonishing array of forms of speech, each one with its own vocabulary, grammar, inflections, and so on?[62]

Central to my proposal is the claim that human beings did not invent languages: languages created themselves. They did so with everything that was required in their own field: their terms (signifiers and meanings [*significados*]), their composition rules, what they lack, and what works as impossible in their specific universe.

As a way of strengthening my argument, it is worth recalling that there is a field not very well known to the general public, but common to several disciplines, such as translation studies, journalism, linguistics, and rhetoric, focused on the study of the "**genius of the language**" [*el genio de la lengua*]. For my project, this is an unavoidable topic, not only because it appears all along Lacan's teaching, but also because it is tightly articulated with "It *(ça)* speaks" and "It *(ça)* enjoys [*jouit*]." When seriously examined (as they should be), these claims entail that languages create themselves. Let us examine this point.

What interests me the most in the expression "genius of language" is that which is introduced by the term "genius," which means, in Latin, the tutelary deity presiding over conception and, therefore, the future. The term has roots in the Indo-European languages, which refer to the following meanings: generate, engender, cause, produce, and form. From the eighth century it has been used to refer to the particular features of a living reality (e.g., the genius of a people, a nation, a country, a language). In Voltaire's *Dictionnaire Philosophique* of 1764, the entry corresponding to the expression starts as follows: "The expression 'genius of language' refers to the language's ability to say, in the shortest and most harmonious way, what in other places is expressed less satisfactorily."[63]

Today, those who are devoted to the study of this fascinating issue claim that "… the genius of language created and keeps creating expressions…."[64] Further,

> …the genius of language is very wise. I ignore what it will decide."[65] Voltaire identifies it with the Muses.[66] Gerardo Vázquez-Ayora describes it as the spirit, the soul, the personality of a language.[67] Alex Grijelmo calls it "the soul of the language.[68]

Émile Benveniste, the renowned linguist, does not make use of the same expression, but argues along the same lines:

> Let us focus our attention on [Aristotle's] six categories in their nature and in their grouping. It seems to us that these predications do not refer to attributes discovered in things, but to a classification arising from the language itself.[69]
>
> Language provides the fundamental configuration of the properties of things as recognized by the mind.[70]

Philologist Victor Klemperer holds,

> But language does not simply write and think for me, it also increasingly dictates my feelings and governs my entire spiritual being the more unquestioningly and unconsciously I abandon myself to it.[71]

And the semiologist Roland Barthes writes,

> But language—the performance of a language system—is neither reactionary nor progressive, it is quite simply fascist; for fascism does not prevent speech, it compels speech.[72]

Lacan makes noteworthy use of the notion of "genius of language." He quotes Albert Dauzat's *Le génie de la langue française* and employs the expression in his writings and seminars from 1946 to 1974. He establishes values and meanings of the genius of language for French, English, German, and Greek. He even claims that the genius of language puts the emphasis where it should go,[73] that it has wonderfully accomplished the role of the "boatswain"[74] entailed by it,[75] and that it constrains,[76] and even creates words.[77]

However, due to the prevalence of Western individualism and substantialism, we are unable to accept that words and expressions are not created by someone or by a plurality of individuals.

No one doubts that one is the author of her own dreams, even when it may well be the case that one is dreamed of—something that the ancient Greeks knew very well.[78] The problem with the prevailing view is that a subject's existence will not be recognized unless one has identified first an individual, in flesh and bones, that ultimately bears responsibility for his utterances, acts, dreams, parapraxes, and symptoms. It is not by chance that Lacan, in one of his last major writings, *L'étourdit*, writes:

> What strikes one at first is to what extent the saidman [*hommodit*] managed to make do with anything coming from the unconscious, until the moment when, by saying it is "structured like a language", I left people thinking that in spite of speaking so much, not much of weight has been said about it: that it/the id chatters, let it chatter, it's all it knows how to do. I have been so little understood so much the better, that I can expect one day that people will raise an objection against me.[79]

We *parlêtres* are "the slaves of language and, still more, of discourse." We are never its masters. We are subjected to the condition of being said: saidmen. Lacan puts it so:

> And the subject, while he may appear to be the slave of language, is still more the slave of a discourse in the universal movement of which his place is already inscribed at his birth, if only in the form of his proper name.[80]

Pain, as well as all other sensations, affections and sentiments, sex,[81] pleasure and displeasure, love and hate, the will, the life and death that we admit, endure, suffer, enjoy, and desire—these are all signifiers. This means they exist as caused by signifiers, and they do so in the form provided by the signifying order and discourse.

Lacan, as he does in many other instances, claims it categorically:

> Men, women, and children are nothing but signifiers.[82]

Naturally, this is not to say that, for instance, the nerve of a damaged wisdom tooth cannot bring about any "pain." However, that we experience pain, the length and the meaning of it—none of this comes from the damaged tissue. And whatever may come purely and exclusively from the latter we cannot know, no matter how many electrodes or scanning devices we hook up to our brains. No biomedical order will ever coincide with the passion of the *parlêtres*: between the damaged nerve and the brain, the big bang of language and discourse has been irrevocably interposed.

We do not feel anything similar to what animals experience, including rats and monkeys. Consider that when someone claims that a dog "feels pain," "is sad" or "is happy," all of this (even the very idea of "feeling") is fundamentally different from what we, as subjects, feel as pain, sadness, or happiness. One should use the term "pain" in both cases only as homonymous. The same applies to all sensation of pleasure, displeasure, satisfaction, appetite, etc.

Although Lacan never managed to articulate his theories to the big bang theory, he established an absolute difference between what comes from the biological body and what comes from language, discourse, and the Other. Indeed, in a remarkable passage referring to instinct and drive, he claims,

> And so I insist on promoting the idea that, whether grounded or not in biological observation, instinct—among the modes of knowledge *[connaissance]* required by nature of living beings so that they satisfy its needs—is defined as a kind of [experiential] knowledge *[connaissance]* we admire because it cannot become [articulated] knowledge *[un savoir]*. But in Freud's work something quite different is at stake, which is a *savoir* certainly, but one that does not involve the slightest *connaissance,* in that it is inscribed in a discourse of which the subject—who, like the messenger-slave of Antiquity, carries under his hair the codicil that condemns him to death—knows neither the meaning nor the text, nor in what language *[langue]* it is written, nor even that it was tattooed on his shaven scalp while he was sleeping.[83]

The *parlêtre* will never be able to know about the instinctual knowledge intrinsic to its nature: it is forgotten. The drive, on the contrary, is a knowledge *[saber]* constituted through the articulation of signifiers, a text inscribed on the body as a message coming from language and discourse.

When it comes to our passions, sensations, and affects, it is imperative to admit that language and discourse operate as a big bang. Only then will we be able to abandon the biological, genetic, and hormonal study of the living substance—red, grey, or white—to start focusing on etymology—the "etymology" of passions—conceived as a discipline where philology, linguistics, history, sociology, anthropology, philosophy, political analysis, ethics, and the sciences of discourse, converge. This is a project otherwise already carried out. Yvonne Bordelois' work comes to mind.[84] It is in the confluence of these different fields, articulated in a way that is particular to psychoanalysis, that it will be possible to raise and examine, among many other issues, the problem of pain and satisfaction in the subject's universe, infinitely foreign to that of the brain, hormones, and genes.

Pain, love, satisfaction, etc., are not at all the same in English, Japanese, Hebrew, or Aymara, and even in each of these languages, they will not be the same in this century as in the previous ones.

When the good clinical medical doctors confront in their practice the difficult, modern problem of chronic pain, they know that Western, modern medicine—a discipline that may be characterized as an attempt to *erase all meaning*[85]—by only considering a purely biological body, cannot explain the cases where pain itself becomes a very complex clinical issue (as we see happening more and more often). Many decades ago, it was already diagnosed that the West suffers from a chronic pandemic of pain. At least since the beginning of the twentieth century, a new clinic emerged: *the clinic of pain*,[86] a new medical specialty that a significant number of patients have already tried to benefit from, often unsuccessfully.

To a great extent, the problem is paradoxical. On the one hand, the West suffers from a pandemic of chronic pain that is getting even worse. On the other, analgesics in these societies are widely available and increase in effectiveness year after year. Even so, the number of patients with chronic pain continues to increase. How is this possible?

Although it may be difficult for many people—especially psychoanalysts—to accept, the reason is not hard to understand: the cause of most forms of pain does not lie in the anatomical body. Further, what affects this body biologically is not effective in reducing the pandemic of chronic pain, which increases suffering even more.

Modern Western culture—extremely individualistic, biologistic, and medicalized—is not only incapable of curing pain, but is also the cause of the increase of pain. This is why medications, even though there is nothing deficient in them at the chemical and biological level, cannot solve the problem. Rather,

> Pain is always personal and always cultural. This is why it is always open to the variable influence of meaning.[87]

Having reached this point in my argument, it is worth remembering the results of the study conducted by Seymour Fisher and Roger Greenberg and published in 1989. The subject-matter of their study was the serious doubts raised by the very poor results of medication for psychological disorders when submitted to rigorous scrutiny, also in the laboratory, when compared with placebo and psychotherapies.[88] Their work showed that in clinical trials there is no significant difference between the therapeutic power of psychotropic medication, placebos, and psychotherapies.

Thus, what biologists, neuroscientists, and other experimental researchers—frequently referred to as "psycho-neuro-immuno-endocrinologists"—call love, hate, pleasure, envy, faith, etc., i.e., the things they claim to find in their research with rats, monkeys, and people, and which they think of as originating in the genes, the immunological system, the hormones, or the brain, are nothing but the result of the improper use of specific effects of the signifier's structure and the locus of the Other. These effects cannot be studied in the laboratory. If this is correct, one should challenge each and every "scientific discovery" mentioned on the following chart:

| | | |
|---|---|---|
| A gene determines male monogamy | Clarín[89] | September 3, 2008 |
| Love and hate share the same brain area | La Nación | October 30, 2008 |
| Cocaine addiction could lie in the genes | Clarín | November 12, 2008 |
| The bigger the brain capacity is, the greater the tendency to lie | Clarín | December, 24, 2008 |
| Kisses are a means to chemically evaluate the romantic compatibility between two people | La Nación | February 14, 2009 |
| Faith lies in a gene | New York Times (Spanish edition) | November 21, 2009 |
| The fear of losing money lies in a brain area | La tercera (Chile) | February 10, 2010 |
| The woman's brain prefers love and hope to having sex | New York Times (Spanish edition) | April 30, 2010 |
| Altruism, decisions regarding one's finances, and political ideas have a genetic basis | Clarín | May 9, 2010 |
| Hormones govern confidence and skepticism | New York Times (Spanish edition) | June 19, 2010 |
| Racial prejudices have a neurological basis | La Nación | November 4, 2010 |
| Lying has its own brain traces | Clarín | October 29, 2010 |
| Friendship is based on a genetic component | Clarín | January 19, 2011 |
| A person's ideology is influenced up to 50% by genetic factors | La Nación | May 27, 2012 |

Affects, such as the sentiments and sensations that, according to these findings, are "localized" or "originated" in the somatic body, do not reside in the tri-dimensional biological body, but only in the bi-dimensional universe of language and discourse. There is an infinite incompatibility between the experimental order and that of the *parlêtres'* lives.[90] Any approach that speaks of "happy brains," "romantic genes," "faithful hormones" should be radically challenged. This is something Lacan did since the beginning of his research. By coining the term "the bias of parallelism,"[91] Lacan criticized Freud because in his model, the "system perception-consciousness" associates an animal, biological term with an effect of the *parlêtres'* language and discourse.

The above-mentioned findings that I am criticizing manifest the development of the biologistic paradigm of the subject, one that has been in existence for several centuries. I will, however, restrict my analysis to some milestones in Western modern history, where the attempt is made to establish that the effects of language, culture, society, and history come from the biological body.

First, consider Edward O. Wilson's research, as presented in his 1975 book, *Sociobiology*, which, based on a Neo-Darwinist evolutionary theory, achieved an alleged "new synthesis."[92] Wilson, one of the most renowned and awarded scientists of the twentieth century, argues that morality comes from the genes, and that all social behavior has its roots in biology, concluding that philosophy must be substituted by biology.

Consider also Richard Dawkins' *The Selfish Gene: The Biological Basis of our Behavior*. In this book, the author argues that biology explains egoism, altruism, love, hate, greed, generosity, and theft. He defines, objectively and univocally, for instance, egoism and well-being in bees, praying mantes, and sea-gulls as established from their "real behavior" and their "action's real effects." He even claims that,

> Yet the chimp feels and thinks and—according to recent experimental evidence—may even be capable of learning a form of human language.[93]

In the context of our discussion, another scientifically prestigious and academically renown professor worth mentioning is Steven Pinker, who, like Wilson, is a Harvard professor and researcher. Pinker has greatly contributed to the advancement of the biologistic paradigm of the subject. In his 1994 book, *The Instinct of Language*, he argues that language is an instinct, taking to an extreme the ideas of his mentor, Noam Chomsky.

Pinker claims that the human brain was modified by natural selection, thereby developing computational microcircuits, from which syntax, morphology, and the lexicon of all languages originate.[94] According to him, language is a human instinct integrated into the brain through an evolutionary process in the same way that spiders weave and birds sing. To claim such a thing, Pinker must defend the notion of the existence of the Universal Language, the Universal Mind, and the Universal People, as they are part of the species.[95] At this point, one may raise the question as to how this was made possible in the first place. Pinker's response: through a genetic mutation. In the case of language, what was created was a first "grammar mutant."[96] In one of the book's chapters, surprisingly entitled, "big bang,"[97] Pinker acknowledges, very reluctantly, the logical problems deriving from the alleged existence of a "first mutant speaking animal:"

> That the first mutant would not have anyone to talk to.
> That the grammar gene has not been found yet.

Finally, not being aware perhaps of the logical consequences of his own claims and contradicting the spirit of his project, Pinker writes, "So human language differs dramatically from natural and artificial animal communication,"[98] and "The first steps toward human language are a mystery,"[99] and finally, "Obviously there is still a huge gulf between these relatively crude systems [the proto-language of homo erectus] and the modern adult language instinct...."[100]

But this is not all, for one could ask too: what is the language spoken by the first speaking animal? The alleged genetic mutation in the brain of the first mutant cannot account for the emergence of a first language. At most, it may justify new "animal" capacities and behaviors, but never the advent of a language.

These are significant problems in his proposal. On top of this, though, this modern, audacious, and famous author includes in his *curriculum vitae*, published on the institutional web page of Harvard's Department of Psychology, a scanned image of his own brain as well as his genome report. His reasons for doing this are evident.[101]

Wilson, Dawkins, and Pinker's arguments aim to sustain a biological project. To accomplish this, they must reduce the signifier to the word, and the latter to the name of things. They also need to omit the difference between meaning [*significado*] and sense [*sentido*], reducing thereby all language to a series of names, meanings (i.e., referred objects), and corresponding compositional laws. Once meaning and sense have been removed from language, it is no longer possible to conceive of jokes, poetry, rhetoric, insults, misunderstandings, flirtatious remarks [*piropos*], lies, etc., i.e., everything that requires interpretation and without which no "natural" language exists.

## Lacan on the Status of Libido, the Drives, and the Body

From an opposing perspective, Lacan, in *Seminar XXIII*—one of his last seminars—criticizes the ways in which different psychoanalytic theories conceive of that which is thought of as being originated in the body, the famous **drives** [*pulsiones*]. Sadly, Lacan's remarks have not been seriously taken into consideration yet.

At this point, it is worth recalling Lacan's stance on the biological body. This is crucial, for, if one does not reconsider the status of the libido, the drives, and *jouissance* in psychoanalysis, these concepts may end up playing the role of securing the biologistic views prevailing in the psychoanalytic domain. If I have criticized these views, it is because I consider psychoanalysis to be precisely that practice that emerged with the aim of curing bodily pains by theoreticizing their cause as belonging to the order of the signifier and the Other.[102]

Lacan's view is clear and it is necessary to stress it: "[Psychoanalysts] do not think that the drives are the echo in the body of the fact that there is a saying."[103] On the contrary, for Lacan, what comes first and lies in the origin, operating as a "fact," is *a saying. A saying* from which drives emerge, which, in turn, fall upon the body in a deceiving manner: they make us believe that they come from its inside, just like the phenomenon of the echo creates the illusion that it is the mountain that is speaking to us.

Thus, what Lacan criticizes is something that Freud believed from the beginning until the end of his theoretical research, despite the fact that it was Freud himself who created for psychoanalytic practice a procedure and a setting [*dispositivo*] built around speech [*la palabra*] and transference, which refutes his own beliefs.

It is on these motives that Lacan established, as a structural fact:

"That one says remains forgotten...".[104]

It is worth clarifying that this is a property established by our society and culture. In other words, it well could be the case that it is not forgotten that one say.

As for how drives are conceptualized, one must confront, on the one hand, the Newtonian and Freudian physical models and, on the other, the relativistic and quantum field theories utilized by Lacan. For Freud, as for Newton, what exists is the energy-endowed tri-dimensional matter and a linear and evolutionary time. In contrast, for the field model integrated into relativity theory, mass and energy are equated and time is not evolutionary.[105] The notion of a body existing in a linear and evolutionary time and invested with energy refers to an already surpassed theoretical model.

Freud defines the libido as an energy originated in the sexual organs' chemism.[106] Lacan, making use of a myth of his own creation, rejects such conception and proposes a conception of the libido as a bi-dimensional surface that, as the *parlêtre's* biological life, escapes.[107]

It is no longer possible to ignore that the drive, understood as the energy transmitted to the psychical apparatus from and by means of the biological body, is rooted in a theory that maintains the existence of a tri-dimensional individual substance invested with energy. In other words, it is a theory assimilated to the model of an intuitive physics.

Lacan thinks of the drive through the following formula: ($ ◊ D). Which of these terms could come from the living substance or account for a somatic energy? Obviously, none.

Other than the big bang, there are several motives for the substitution of the Newtonian physical model used by Freud for the relativistic and quantum physics models. According to the latter—this is a thesis entirely agreed upon by scientists—observation modifies the phenomenon being observed, something that can be rendered as a genuine principle: observing a system modifies the system.[108] Or better yet: "observation actually *creates* the observed physical reality."[109]

This principle provides us with an appropriate logical model to conceive of the clinic as a *transferential* clinic sustained by the analyst's desire. It should be noted that the latter is a concept proposed by Lacan to rectify the Freudian notion of the observing analyst's neutrality as that which secures the scientific character of psychoanalysis.

We have to admit that reality as such does not exist prior to its observation. The same principle applies in the psychoanalytic clinic.

Another principle of quantum mechanics should be highlighted: the uncertainty principle mentioned by Lacan in his seminar of May 25, 1955. In his lecture, Lacan claims that each time something that belongs to the order of language is manifested, it is inevitable that the quantum physics' uncertainty principle comes into play:

It is clear that it's in relation to language that something funny happens. That is what Heisenberg's principle [the uncertainty principle] comes down to.

When one is in a position to determine one of the properties of the system, one cannot formulate the others. When one speaks of the location of electrons, when one tells them to stay put somewhere, to remain always in the same place, one loses all sense of what is commonly called their velocity. Conversely, if one tells them—well then, alright, you must always move in the same way—one no longer has any idea where they are. I am not saying that we will always be in this eminently ludicrous position. But until things change, we can say that the elements do not answer where one asks them. More precisely, if one asks them somewhere, it is impossible to grasp them as a whole.[110]

My general criticism of empirical research projects is that they omit the uncertainty principle posited by every use of the terms of a language and believe, accordingly, that these terms can be isolated as if they were corpuscles.[111] Further, in the psychoanalytic clinic, the uncertainty principle provides us with the tools needed to admit what Lacan called, "the analyst's nescience," i.e., the structural impossibility of knowing what is meant and entailed by the signifiers at play in a clinical case until they have been articulated, in a conjectural form, in their corresponding network [*red*].

The previously listed reports on the most modern scientific research in neurology, endocrinology, and genetics are rooted in a widespread confusion that today, paradoxically, has attained the status of a genuine paradigm, one that enjoys popular acceptance.

In bio-laboratories, there is the belief that one can work with what is supposed to be faithfulness, hate, love, lies, fear, generosity, hope, altruism, trust, skepticism, etc., by reducing them to their univocal, isolated, and implicit definitions. Accordingly, this kind of research could not be but highly biased. Because polysemy and context are excluded from the way those terms are used, the cultural, historical, social, linguistic, discursive, and particular differences are also left aside.

## Modern Physics, Philosophy, Psychoanalysis, and Our Ordinary Image of "Reality"

At this point in my argument, it is worth introducing some philosophical reflections on these problems. Western philosophy, born in Greece, emerged as a speculation tightly linked to physics and mathematics. However, as a rule, Western philosophy in the last centuries tends to disregard the scientific findings that do not seem intuitively right.

There are some noteworthy exceptions, though. For instance, at the beginning of the twentieth century, what used to be known as the Berlin Circle (which included the already mentioned H. Reichenbach), along with the Vienna Circle, defended a fervent empiricism, preventing thereby the transcendental application of the new concepts of the twentieth-century physics, in their philosophical aspects, to their "scientific philosophy." Their staunch empiricism could not advance the true philosophical subversion they were seeking, for although they worked with the findings of modern physics, they could not do without the empiricist paradigm sustained by their ontology, according to which being is and non-being is not. However, in the twentieth-century physics, phenomena are not observed as the result of looking at corpuscles through a microscope. "Observation" means probabilistic intervention and "observed" entities are, in fact, mathematical conventions. Since the beginning of the last century physics rejects "being is" and "non-being is not."[112]

With the relative exceptions of Alain Badiou and Quintin Meillassoux,[113] who sustain their philosophical work with reference to modern mathematics, twentieth and twenty-first-century philosophers do not tend to consider the paradigm shift in our conceptions of matter, energy, time, and space, i.e., in our accounts of reality and the real, brought about by relativistic, quantum, and string physics. Since Einstein, though, the physicists who created these subversive conceptions have published popular-science books about their discoveries, aiming to articulate the latter along with Western philosophy and show the deep philosophical and ideological transformations required by these discoveries.

W. Heisenberg, to mention a notable example, published *Physics and Philosophy* in the mid-50s. In this work he examines the transformations of the world and ontology necessitated by modern science. Also, today, the physicists Hawking and Mlodinow title the first two chapters of their recent book "The mystery of being" and "What is reality?"

To present the great philosophical transformations caused by modern physics, I selected two quotations. The first is by Einstein and Infeld:

> During the second half of the nineteenth century new and revolutionary ideas were introduced into physics; they opened the way to a new philosophical view, differing from the mechanical one. The results of the work of Faraday, Maxwell, and Hertz led to the development of modern physics, to the creation of new concepts, forming a new picture of reality.[114]

The second quotation is from Argentinean researcher A. Gangui:

> In special relativity, time and space were no longer absolute and mutually independent as Newton thought, but they were combined with each other in the specific manner prescribed by Einstein's theory. This and other discoveries (...) would shatter the foundations of physics to the point that their consequences would surpass the boundaries of science and have a philosophical impact.[115]

On a rational and experimental basis, contemporary physical theories must claim that matter, energy, and the space-time emerge together out of a vacuum or nothingness:[116] how could this not be philosophically relevant? Or is it that philosophy has nothing to say about these issues? Mathematics is based on the notion that one emerges out of zero. Does not this alter our philosophical conceptions? It does not seem so, for as a rule, it is assumed and admitted that one comes first, then two, and that matter is three-dimensional, substantial, tangible, and visible.

We are faced with new realities that alter our metaphysical and ontological conceptions, realities that have been with us for over a century and remain ignored by most philosophers and the general public. It is true that this new "scientific reality" is not intuitive, but why should philosophy be intuitive in the first place?

Further, one of the most severe criticisms of the mathematized sciences raised by the social sciences, and specially psychoanalysis, that encourages the tendency to reject formal paradigms is built around an already outdated argument, namely, that these paradigms aim for a complete explanation of everything. Today, the mathematized sciences are fundamentally characterized by their having contributed to the notion of an unsurpassable boundary, an impossibility. Thus, for instance, they fully recognize and work with the contradiction between the relativistic and the quantum models. Also, loop theory admits millions, perhaps infinite solutions. In the field of mathematics, the Gödel theorem posits an impossibility intrinsic to natural numbers. None of these disciplines proceeds from, or aims to achieve, complete explanations or presupposes that its domain is a complete whole, even when it is usually the case that scientists working in these disciplines take this route.

Another problem that occupies a central place in modern physics that shows unambiguously that science does not work with, or base hypotheses on, complete and coherent "wholes," is that of wave-particle duality, a key component in the scientific account of the real. This account is generally ignored by modern philosophical schools and the general public. Lacan integrated it into his teaching, but his followers did not adequately consider it.

Wave-particle or wave-corpuscle duality is an apparent paradox that over decades has become an essential concept indisputably accepted by the scientific community. It affirms that in quantum mechanics there are no fundamental differences between waves (being extended in space and without a mass, overlapping and interfering with each other) and particles (occupying an exclusive and precise place in space and having a mass). This has been a polemical issue in the context of the discussion on the nature of light since the mid-seventeenth century. At that time, two theories about light predominated: Christian Huygens' wave theory and Isaac Newton's corpuscular theory. As expected, given the prevailing substantialist and empiricist prejudices, the latter was upheld for almost two centuries. Today we know that light (electromagnetic waves observable to the human eye) has a nature unsuspected by common sense: depending on how it is posited, light will be a wave (a light beam) or a particle (a photon). The issue is, however, much wider: everything can have wave or particle-like properties, depending on how it is observed. Precisely because it poses an epistemological obstacle, this has been described as the major enigma of quantum physics and its best-kept secret.[117]

If this is the picture offered to us by modern science, perhaps we should raise the question as to whether psychoanalysis itself works with a complete paradigm of universal scope. A psychoanalysis that rejects the most subversive theses of Lacan's teaching is doomed to go in exactly this direction.

As expected, given the fundamental character of these scientific issues, Lacan, in his continuous study and articulation of psychoanalysis with modern, mathematized physics, was aware of its surprising theory of the real and its consequences for our conception of the subject. For instance, in *Seminar XVII, Psychoanalysis upside-down*, he argues,

> …the division of the subject is something quite different. If "where he is not, he is thinking," and if "where he is not thinking, he is," it is precisely because he is in both places. I would even say that this formula of the *Spaltung* is improper. The subject participates in the real precisely in that it is apparently impossible. Or, to put it better, if I had to employ a figure that does not occur here by chance, I would say that the case with it is like that of the electron, where the latter is posited as being at the intersection of wave theory and corpuscular theory. We are forced to admit that it is as one and the same that it passes through two distant holes at the same time. Thus, the order of what we represent as the *Spaltung* of the subject is different from the one that determines that truth can only be represented by being stated only in a half-saying.[118]

The subject is therefore posited as being related to one of the most surprising and anti-intuitive properties of the electron. Indeed, on the issue of the wave-particle duality, quantum physics claims that an electron "is a particle" or "is a wave" depending on the observer.

Both the uncertainty principle and the wave-particle duality—properties that among others, characterize the profound subversion that physics since the beginning of the nineteenth century entails for our conception of the material universe— were integrated by Lacan into his psychoanalytic theory. We know that they require a deep, radical shift in the current model used to characterize matter, energy, time, and space, but what are the consequences of thinking of the subject along the axes of the wave-particle duality?

In Lacan's teaching, the subject will be a function of how it is posited: as a particle (a corpuscle) or as a wave (a motion). If the former, it will occupy a place in space, have a mass, and will be posited as a *parlêtre*; if the latter, it will interfere with other waves, which always overlap and lack mass. Further, it will be in two different places at the same time. The latter is what Lacan presented as the split of the subject. None of this has anything to do with the half-saying, the ineffable, or with Freud's splitting of psychic personality into ego, super-ego, and *id*.

This is, then, what Lacan presents as the subject's division at the end of his teaching. Thus, whether the clinic centers around a flesh-and-bones **body** or a **wave** susceptible of being interfered with and intertwined in an inmixing of alterity depends on the psychoanalyst. Only the second option allows an *in*-transference-clinic, exclusive to psychoanalysis.

## The Big Bang and the Biologistic Paradigms

When it comes to the interpretation of the subject and all its specific phenomena, I suggest—along with criticism of the naïve, vulgar, and prejudiced conceptions of the reality of bodies—that psychoanalysis must work with the notion of a "biological forgetfulness." If we follow this line of thought, what seems to originate in the animal body will be seen as caused by the big bang of language and the social link established by particular discourses. Thus, in psychoanalysis and all the social disciplines, among which medicine is partially included, all bodily manifestations are signifying and entail meanings not susceptible to definition except through a linguistic and contextual interpretation.

What is enjoyable or painful, satisfying or unpleasant, no longer belongs to the world of nature, because what came from the latter in a pure state has been forever forgotten. Although this stance fully admits that bacteria and viruses can make the biological body sick, it stresses that one should always reflect upon complaints about suffering and pain in the medical or psychoanalytic clinic by accepting the big bang of language and discourse.

Let us now consider a series of examples that clearly illustrate the opposition between the biologistic and the big bang paradigms.

Neurology takes lying to be associated with the size of the brain; Lacan thinks of it as the gravitational law of discourse.[119] If one can lie, as everyone knows, by saying, "I am heading to Krakov," so my interlocutor believes I am heading to Lemberg, when in fact I am indeed heading to Krakov then one can tell a lie by speaking the truth, as the most superficial reflection on the bluff shows, not only in poker, but in the domain of economy, politics, and virtually every social situation. In what area of the brain should one seek it? Is the one responsible for our truths or the one responsible for our lies? Is there a brain area corresponding to true truths, even though they do not exist? Did the scientists who participated in this neurological research consider the liar paradox? According to brain studies, is Epimenides telling the truth or is he lying?

In the signifying universe nothing is in itself, as each signifier only is what others are not. As truths may not be true, no term can be identical to itself, neither the signifiers nor its effects. This is why, in this view, true truth, loving love, and hateful hate are eradicated. Truth, love, hate, etc., structurally require a system of at least four signifying terms to occupy a position in their corresponding place, i.e., in a chain of discourse and in reference to all other articulated signifiers.

For example, say I discover that I loved someone after being told so by others, despite never having felt it, and 20 years after leaving her. This is something that could happen to anyone. If so, how could this love be located in the brain, the genes, or hormones? School children, not yet contaminated by the paradigm criticized here, claim that "those who fight love each other." Could our current scientists, in their laboratory work, make proper sense of such a claim? For some, love is a "game of give and take." For Lacan, as he claims throughout his teaching, love is "to give what one does not have." In Plato's famous *Symposium*, one finds different conceptions of love; today, there is the popularized notion of a "liquid love."

Which among these different accounts of love are found in the experiments of neuroscientists and geneticists? All of them—even when they are so different and, in some cases, contradict one another? Where would psycho-neuro-immuno-endocrinology localize the love of German Romanticism—one that so strongly models how we Westerners feel—a love tightly linked to death, even if it is not lived this way in other cultures?

This problem is not solved by consulting the experiments' "subjects." The notion of unconscious in psychoanalysis, as I understand it, warns us that one's opinion is no longer admissible as a justification for one's stance. The primordial psychoanalytic truth is that the I (what I think and what I feel) does not coincide with what *It* thinks and *It* enjoys [Sp. *goza*; Fr. *jouit*].

Another crucial example is **faith**. India's religious world is populated by hundreds of deities: is there in India a modality of faith comparable to the prevailing, millenary monotheisms of the West? And even within the "schemes" that sustain Western monotheisms, is Christian faith the same thing as the Hebrew *emuná*? To which of these do the scientific studies publicized in the mass media refer? Are they aware that this last question has no unique answer, but many, each of them opposing and contradicting all others? Christianity, for instance, rationally responds to specific questions, whereas Judaism rejects the act of questioning. In other words, in one case one must respond with a "yes," while in the other, one is not supposed to raise questions at all. More broadly, is religion a similar phenomenon in the West, Asia, and Africa?

As for **everyday habits**, M. Mauss was the first to propose that the most "natural" ways of eating, drinking, walking, sitting, having intercourse, etc., are strictly social and cultural. In a similar vein, one must accept, P. Bourdieu's proposal that there is even a "social sense of taste," not only in its aesthetic aspect, but also in relation to flavors: the qualities "savoury," "sour," "delicious," or "rancid" are not natural for the *parlêtre*.

Finally, consider the case of **pain**. The key question on this issue is, what can laboratory experimental studies say about the pain that provides pleasure and is sought out? Would this also count as "pain"? If I enjoy that it hurts, even if I am not aware of this enjoyment, where should the electrodes be put, on the locus of the pain or the pleasure? And what is enjoyed with a particular someone but experienced as pain with another person, in what part of the tangible body could this be originated? Vaginal delivery is painful, but not in all cultures and times—this is the question.

Let me stress that the position I am advocating does not deny the fact that, for instance, Down's and Turner syndromes are genetic pathologies. They are, and this is precisely why one can establish a series of typical effects of these pathologies. Obviously, I am not suggesting that they are caused by the register of the signifier and the Other. However, one must reject that in each particular case these pathologies bring about unhappiness, sadness, joy, etc. Rather, these terms belong—we can use again the reference to cosmology—to *another* universe. If in any of these cases, issues of love, envy, or anger emerged, then one would have to consider that the ones affected are *parlêtres* and that the big bang of language and discourse has already been operative, having interposed itself between the genetic disease and the signifying effects.

There are cases where it may be difficult to decide whether a particular genetic, hormonal, or neurological pathology is a consequence of a biological disease or of the order of language and discourse. These ambiguous cases exist and should not be dismissed. My stance regarding such cases is to sustain doubt, to raise and keep open the question, "Could it be that the pathology is 'to some extent,' 'also,' or even 'for the most part' caused by the signifier and the Other?" This is a question that one hears less and less frequently in the consulting rooms of doctors, psychologists, and psychoanalysts.

Psychoanalysts, as the professionals criticized earlier and society as a whole, embrace the biologistic paradigm. Armed with a heavily naturalistic logic, they claim that the biological body is the real, despite the fact that what Lacan posits is that the real is the logically and mathematically impossible [*lo imposible lógico-matemático*]. For him, this is an account of the real that is the basis of modern physics.

The spirit of our time and the prevailing ideas in our society and culture make it difficult for such an account to be accepted. I will illustrate this by means of reference to two eminent authors in the Lacanian field. Gerard Pommier, one of Lacan's famous patients and disciples, published a book where he posits the existence of neurotransmitters for *jouissance*,[120] as if Lacan's *jouissance* could lie in biological entities. For him, the latter exists in a meaningful and sense-less manner: they "simply are." On the other hand, Jacques-Alain Miller, Lacan's son-in-law and editor and the most influential psychoanalytic author today, claims that *jouissance* is autistic and the most singular thing in each of us, originating in our biological body.[121] These are surprising claims. In fact, Lacan, from the beginning to the end of his elaboration of *jouissance*, never ceased to link it, in an essential manner, to meaning [*sentido*]. For instance, he claimed:

…to render *jouissance* possible is the same thing as what I will write: *j'ouis-sens*. It is the same thing as to hear a meaning.[122]

Miller's assertions are even more puzzling insofar as Lacan maintained, especially at the end of his teaching, that *jouissance* exists as jA (jouissance of the Other and therefore not one's own) and jφ (a phallic *jouissance* irreducible to the boundaries of the body). Undoubtedly, neither of these is a *jouissance* of the flesh. As a consequence: (a) neurotransmitters of *jouissance* cannot exist (*jouissance* is beyond the body) and (b) there cannot be an autistic *jouissance* (*jouissance* is always of the Other).

## Particularity, Singularity, and the Concept of Subject

There is an important problem left. If language and the Other exist before the individual biological body is born, where do particular differences come from, the existence of such differences being one of the major pillars upon which psychoanalytic practice is built?

Regarding particular differences (later I will address the issue of their cause), I posit a distinction between "singular" and "particular." Today it is claimed, especially in the field of Lacanian psychoanalysis, that the "subject is singular." The meanings of "particular" and "singular," both in French and in English, partially overlap. This is an issue that cannot be avoided in an essay on the big bang, which is precisely *the* singularity of the universe or, equivalently, *the* singularity of mathematical-physics, i.e., the point where the theory collapses because it implies the notion of an infinite quantity of energy.

"Singular" refers to the isolated, the unique, the rare, and the extraordinary, while "particular" points to that which, remaining different from everything other than itself, is established only in relation to and as a function of the Other. The former favors the individual and the exception; the latter, participation in relation to and as a distinctive part of a structure. In Lacan's account of the subject, the particular condition of its existence is asserted as *pars*,[123] i.e., as a "part" of a structure, in such a way that the singular condition is rejected: for Lacan, there is "no subject without the Other" and the two are in a relation of inmixing.[124]

The prevailing assumption in psychoanalysis is that the singular condition originates in the biological body. É. Durkheim puts it this way: "there must be a factor of individuation; it is the body that plays this role."[125] This view is also asserted by Freud in his accounts of lived experiences of satisfaction and dissatisfaction and their corresponding mnemic singular traces. For Freud, all of this is indubitable. Many contemporary Lacanians speak of "each one's singular *jouissance*." However, there are many sources that comprise a particular condition. If we return to the earlier distinctions that helped us circumscribe Lacan's concept of subject, it is clear that all of them contribute to the generation of individuality, as shown in the following table:

| Instantiations [of the field of language and discourse] | Field | Individual condition |
| --- | --- | --- |
| Individual | The biological domain | DNA, finger prints, etc. |
| Person | The realm of history and society | A person is determined by chronological time, geographical place, etc. |
| Citizen | The legal and political realm | Passport, etc. |

One should not rely on the notion that singular differences originate in the biological body, stemming from the "living substance" and the exclusive experiences it underwent since its birth. Unless biological traits and differential experiences, as functions of language and its Other, mean something for someone, pure biological data does not change by itself either the meaning [*significado*] or the sense [*sentido*] of life. If they do, they inaugurate the beyond of all saying: the field of sense.[126] In this case, traits operate as signifiers, not as natural signals. If, for instance, one's height or skin color connotes the sense and meaning of life, then they operate as signifiers in the chain of discourse and are, consequently, invested with the values that those elements had and still have for others and the Other in the signifying context and the social, cultural, religious, and linguistic universe, which is where we genuinely live.

From this perspective, which I see as a necessary development of Lacan's most subversive stance—his subversion of the subject—three important remarks are in order:

1  Precisely as a consequence of his reflection on these issues regarding particularity, Lacan, by means of a neologism, deemed it necessary to develop a new concept: *lalangue*, which establishes the field of the particular coordinates of a *parlêtre's* relation to a "mother tongue." This is not a problem one finds in linguistic research. It indicates *lalangue's* ineliminable coordination with the mother tongue, understanding by the latter the value and meanings given by the particular and the family history in each case, condensed in terms of the signifying battery in their corresponding network—terms that usually do not belong to a single natural language.
2  Each subject occupies the empty place between two signifiers, which, besides being in a relation of mutual articulation, are distinguished from all others within a structure and contribute to the articulated network of several signifying chains. All of this, clearly, is a particular formation.
3  The subject also occupies a particular place in the chain or braid of discourse in that this place articulates the historical interweaving of signifying relationships (such as family institutions) among the members of at least three generations: those who have been integrated as a grandchild, son, brother, father, adopted son, etc. This integration assigns to each *parlêtre* a particular place within a tight structure.

Each of the particular articulations of these places located between the signifiers and the chains or braids of discourse is named, by Lacan, "subject;" I propose the term, **"intervallic subject."**[127]

The structure of these intervals—the intervallic subject—is not already definitively fixed, and because it operates according to the logic of a circular time, the structure is not like a fate or an inevitable future. However, it is characterized by its being widely determined as a particular structure with causal powers (none of which includes the brain, genes, or hormones), allowing only new, signifying acts as a function of terms that already operate according to the logic [*sentido*] of the structure, terms that have specific values provided by the others and the Other. This is why, in this account, the idea of freedom is rejected. The new can certainly emerge, but only as a function of the coordinates of its own context in the modality of the tense called "future perfect."

When in a 1972 television interview Lacan was asked about the relation between freedom and psychoanalysis—an issue highly valued by those psychoanalysts who base their stance on the idea of subjective responsibility—he laughingly replied: "Yes…, those terms…, they make me laugh, yes…, I never speak of freedom."[128]

One can be a creator, a revolutionary, or even a subversive individual. One can create terms, objects, and practices, all of them new—something that takes place often in societies like ours that advocate change and progress. It is impossible, though, that these things happen beyond the boundaries of the linguistic, religious, ideological, familiar, and political realms, among others. Not even scientists can make discoveries or inventions that go beyond the theoretical context of their time. It would have been impossible, for instance, for Einstein's theories—though they are among the most surprising cases of creativity and novelty brought about by a single person—to exist before topology, Brownian motion theory, the light quantum hypothesis, and the paradoxes within the measurements of the speed of light. The "theory of relativity" was simultaneously discovered, albeit in different orientations, by A. Einstein and H. Poincaré,[129] which demonstrates that these discoveries depended more on theoretical developments in the scientific and intellectual contexts than on the particular conditions of these individual scientists.

## Psychoanalysis and String Theory

At this point it is convenient to make a final connection, this time between psychoanalysis and string theory.[130] I think this is justified in that string theory is a particularly important development in recent physics, but also in that Lacan has a theory of loops, knots, and braids that his followers tend to misinterpret as referring to nylon strings or metal chains, when Lacan, through this theory, is actually positing the function of the hole. The confusion is due to their ignorance of such scientific developments and of Lacan's philosophical stance—his rejection of ontology and his epistemological defense of "conjectural sciences" (a category that includes psychoanalysis). It is also prompted by the prevailing materialistic and substantialist ideology of our time.

String theory is based on quantum physics, for which, according to one interpretation, matter is not composed of particles considered as corpuscles, but of waves. A wave function—a mathematical function, i.e., a genuinely mass-less body, but an "object" of physics nonetheless—consists in crests and valleys and is itself an object to be handled mathematically. For string theory, the wave is the only elementary object.[131] Bojowald writes,

> What may also seem counterintuitive is the interrelation of different objects described by wave functions. While classical particles can be put at separate places like billiard balls, and hit at different speeds to watch their motion and collisions, a single wave function already occupies all of space. (…) Just the presence of the first wave function, anywhere in the universe, has a certain influence on another wave function.[132]

This theory coincides with the manner in which the subject's mode of existence must be conceived, i.e., not as an individual, substantial object (an epiphenomenon of the biological body), invested with energy (libido, drives, or *jouissance*), but as an entity that, without losing its particular condition, exists only in a relation of inmixing, interference, and superposition with others and the Other. In order to understand and accept this, one must drop the ancient Newtonian model, acknowledging not only the current scientific model, but also a new philosophical standpoint, a new image of reality,[133] not populated by tri-dimensional individuals, but by mutually intertwined incorporeal entities.[134]

Reichenbach depicts it as follows:

> There exists no normal system for the interpretation of the unobservables, and we cannot speak of unobservables in the same sense as is implied for the world of everyday life. We can regard the elementary constituents of matter as particles or waves...[135]

From this perspective I hold, with Lacan, that

1   our relation to Otherness is one of inmixing;
2   *It* speaks, thinks, and enjoys [*goza*];
3   there is no reality prior to the social link;
4   the subject is intervallic and, being particular, it is neither individual nor singular.

Continuing this criticism of the old individualistic and substantialist accounts, it is worth reflecting on this passage from Einstein and Infeld:

> The old mechanical view attempted to reduce all events in nature to forces acting between material particles. (...) The recognition of the new concepts grew steadily, until substance was overshadowed by the field. (...) A new reality was created, a new concept for which there was no place in the mechanical description.[136]

Lacan began his teaching by grounding it in the mathematical concept of function and in a notion of field he borrowed from modern physics (cf. *Function and Field of Speech and Language in Psychoanalysis*). How many more decades are needed to consider this seriously and rescue the most original aspects of his contributions from oblivion?

If one favors a transferential clinic (in contraposition to the classical doctor/patient relationship), if one holds the unconscious as the Other's discourse, the subject as existing always immixed with Otherness, and a notion of reality as necessarily preceded by the social link, should not one then cease to take Newton's physics (in its popularized version) as a point of reference? It is not the case that there is reality and then, beside it, science: we dwell in a reality conceived and experienced according to the scientific model that we hold, regardless of our being aware of it or not.

On material reality, Einstein and Infeld write:

> A new concept appears in physics, the most important invention since Newton's time: the field. It needed great scientific imagination to realize that it is not the

charges and the particles but the field in the space between the charges and the particles which is essential for the description of physical phenomena.[137]

And Reichenbach formulates it as follows:

> The experiences offered by atomic phenomena make it necessary to abandon the idea of a corporeal substance...[138]

Thus, the field and wave-function theories, constituting the necessary basis for the development of modern physics, oblige us to revise the issue of the existence of individual entities, particularly those that are to be considered by psychoanalysts. Only then will we be able to advance a distinction between the subject and the individual and determine that which, in the psychoanalytic clinic, counts as a case. According to the logic of fields and waves, elementary matter does not behave as billiard balls colliding on a table do. The latter exemplifies the standard manner in which Western ideology conceives of the way of being of subjects and electrons. The different elements, taken in isolation, participate in a reality that precludes all forms of individualism, for instance, that of Aristotle and Newton's physics, which, in turn, constitute the theoretical foundations of Freud's approach to psychoanalytic cases. In contrast, modern physicists claim that

> Classical theories such as Newton's are built upon a framework reflecting everyday experience, in which material objects have an individual existence, can be located at definite locations, follow definite paths, and so on. Quantum physics provides a framework for understanding how nature operates on atomic and subatomic scales, but (...) it dictates a completely different conceptual schema, one in which an object's position, path, and even its past and future are not precisely determined.[139]

Lacan's work is contemporary with these scientific developments. In his teaching we find a conception of the subject that is in agreement with them, as he posits that the psychoanalytic subject must be considered in a relation of inmixing with Otherness, which entails that "there is no subject without an Other." Further, it means that nothing can be posited as exclusive to "a" singular or individual subject, because in his teaching the term subject is used precisely to reject the individual being. His stance is radical in that it does not posit an individual subject that would *then* be affected by the Other. When one is considering a subject, one is obliged to acknowledge that distinguishing between what belongs to the subject and what belongs to the Other is impossible. Thus, in the psychoanalytic clinic, it is not possible to distinguish between what is said by the analyst and what is said by the analysand. Indeed, *It* speaks, *It* thinks, and *It* enjoys between them and independently of their egos.

By the end of his teaching, Lacan does not deny or abandon his initial stance, grounded on the notions of function and field; quite the contrary, he doubles down. These two quotations suffice to verify this:

The space in which the creations of science are deployed can only be qualified henceforth as the *in-substance,* as the *a-thing, l'achose* with an apostrophe—a fact that entirely changes the meaning of our materialism.[140]

It is in this *moterialism*, if you will allow me to use this word for the first time, that the unconscious takes hold.[141]

This criticism of substantialism and materialism, which passed from Newton's physics to the human and social sciences and posits the existence of tri-dimensional entities loaded with energy, entities that occupy an exclusive place in space at a given moment, had already been raised by some authors working in disciplines close to psychoanalysis. I have in mind especially the work of Norbert Elias, who posited the human as a "mesh fabric" and conceptualized its mode of existence as an "intertwinement:"

...the vision of an irreducible wall between one human being and all others, between inner and outer worlds, evaporates to be replaced by a vision of an incessant and irreducible intertwining of individual beings...[142]

In modern physics, Einstein and Infeld put it this way:

In Maxwell's theory [one of the most important starting points of relativistic physics] there no material actors.[143]

As a result of the arguments I have been proposing, one may claim that for every single psychoanalytic concept and for every single clinical case and its problems there are, fundamentally, two paradigmatic ways of approaching them:

1  What happens in each case is posited as having originated in the individual biological body that, once it is born, confronts the Other, culture, society, history, and a language that will partially alter it. There will be a biological remnant, though: the drives or *jouissance*.
2  From the very beginning there is a signifying structure and the Other, "prior" to everything that may be considered as natural, biological, and individual. As a consequence, for every symptom, phantasy [*fantasma*], desire, drive, *jouissance*, etc., what was once a biological reality has definitively fallen into oblivion as a result of the big bang of language and the Other.

If one accepts the second paradigm, then one must conclude that after the **big bang**, everything that takes place as if it were "coming from the biological body"—the very issue and the subject-matter of psychoanalysis and the other social sciences—does not and cannot come from it: this is only an appearance.

Psychoanalysts must confront the dilemma: do the drives and *jouissance* originate in "the living substance" or are they creations of the signifying structure and the Other? Psychoanalysis could only remain in existence if the latter alternative is defended with reasonable and logically valid arguments that keep up with contemporary scientific debates. Otherwise, the fate of psychoanalysis is disappearance into the field of the so-called psychotherapies and life coaching techniques.

## The Great Chain of Being and the Big Bang of Language and Discourse

The notion that there is a continuity among all beings is one widely accepted since the ancient Greek philosophers. They posited a natural hierarchical scale of material substances starting from the "lowest" inanimate matter gradually leading to the most developed entities and divine beings at the top. Until the eighteenth century, Western culture kept in place the conception of an absolute gap within the "great chain of being"[144] (what I think of as a big bang), a gap that firmly separated human beings from animals. From then on, a new ontological taxonomy emerged and this distinction started to dilute: the task was now to establish which were the missing links needed to rebuild the continuity required by the prevailing scientific views at that time. As a consequence, a process that would degrade human singularity while looking for those "missing links" in the great chain of being was set in motion.

This enterprise finally arrived at the idea that human beings are merely natural animals, and thus are an object of study for zoology.[145]

Thus, the ideological interpretation of science that, as previously described in this book, currently posits the necessity of substituting philosophy and ethics with neurological, genetic, and hormone research gains pace, justifying itself through the notion that "human beings" are barely different than chimpanzees, bonobos, rats, etc., which are purportedly located only a tiny step below humans in the biological order.[146]

It is worth recalling that from this intellectual movement a new "science" emerged, one that goes against reason and, affirming itself as spiritual and intuitive, reestablishes boundaries and differences, but this time among the races. An eminent example of this is, of course, the case of the Nazis, who posited a human race (the Aryan one) as opposed to all others, for instance the Blacks and Jews, conceiving these as races of humans degraded to the category of animals.

In the history of ideas, one always finds that different views are mixed and that many of them have integrated elements from other views. For instance, despite their ideological belief in the gap between the races, even the Nazis felt obligated to defend the existence of a "vital force" internal to all matter. Thus, they are also part of the movement that Rosa Sala Rose describes as an "atrociously materialistic perception," one that ends up embracing a monistic, unifying conception that posits one sole substance and rejects "Descartes' error" of defending an ontological dualism.[147]

This materialist and vitalistic evolutionism is still with us, this time imbued with the alleged "authority of science." This notion of "science" must be entirely reconsidered. For this trend of thought, all knowledge has its origin in the nervous system. As a consequence, they argue, the neurosciences and the biologically-grounded forms of psychology are to substitute all "non-naturalized" forms of epistemology, understanding by "naturalized epistemology"[148] a phase in the development of biology itself. This view is, then, radically opposed to the idea that *It* thinks, *It* speaks, and *It* enjoys.

Regrettably, psychoanalysis, even from its very beginnings, is part of this tendency. Indeed, the influence of the biological theories of Lamarck, Haechel,[149] and others on Freud's views is noticeable and explicitly held even in late texts such as "Moses and Monotheism,"[150] but also in the popular "Lacanian biology" of J.-A. Miller,[151] which is a version of a vitalistic, monistic ontology with "jouissance" at its center.

By proposing a big bang of language and discourse, I intend to provide Lacanian psychoanalytic theory with modern scientific theories that are drawn not from biology, but from physics. Lacan's theory, starting from Cartesian dualism, does not reduce the subject, as Lacanian psychoanalysts tend to do, to a monistic ontology. Quite the contrary, he posits the notion of an "enjoying substance" [*substancia gozante*], entirely anti-ontological in nature, that breaks the chain of being by establishing the subject's lack-in-being [*falta-en-ser*]. Thus, Lacan argues for a materialism—*motérialism*—of language and discourse, in such a way that the specificity of a practice that deals with the *parlêtre* is secured. Given the current state of affairs, not thinking of the subject in these terms and according to this logic favors the most atrocious and murderous forms of racism, xenophobia, and social and sexist discriminatory practices, allegedly justified by differences existing among biological bodies.[152]

## Notes

1   Hereafter, "Other" (capitalized "O") is to be understood as referring to both the battery and the treasure of the signifiers as well as to its historical embodiment.

2   See Eidelsztein, Alfredo, "Diagnosticar el sujeto," in *Imago Agenda* (Buenos Aires: Letra Viva, 2003), p. 73.

3   This neologism coined by Lacan conjugates *parler* (to speak) and *être* (being). Eidelsztein's reading stresses the former over the latter, paving the way for a radically non-individualistic and de-substantialized notion of "subject" [TN].

4   Lacan, Jacques, *Seminar XI*, session of 01.22.1974. In Miller's edition of this seminar, this section is entitled, "The Freudian Unconscious and Ours."

5   Lacan, Jacques, "Position of the Unconscious," in *Écrits* (New York: Norton, 2006), p. 704/830, translation modified. [The second pagination number refers to the original French version of the *Écrits*, the first to the English edition. When, as in this case, I have modified the English translation a passage by Lacan to make it closer to Eidelsztein's quotation of the Spanish version, "translation modified" is added next to my rendition of the passage; *Translator's Note.*]

6   Lacan, Jacques, "Position of the Unconscious," in *Écrits* (New York: Norton, 2006), p. 708/835 [translation modified].

7   Lacan, Jacques, "Position of the Unconscious," in *Écrits* (New York: Norton, 2006), p. 708/835 [translation modified].

8   Lacan, Jacques, "Position of the Unconscious," in *Écrits* (New York: Norton, 2006), p. 712/840.

9   Lacan, Jacques, "Position of the Unconscious," in *Écrits* (New York: Norton, 2006), p. 708/835.
10  Lacan, Jacques, "Position of the Unconscious," in *Écrits* (New York: Norton, 2006), p. 711/839.
11  Lacan, Jacques, *Seminar III*, section XIV, "The Signifier, as such, signifies nothing."
12  Lacan, Jacques, "Position of the Unconscious," in *Écrits* (New York: Norton, 2006), p. 715/843.
13  Lacan, Jacques, "The Subversion of the Subject and the Dialectics of Desire in the Freudian Unconscious," in *Écrits* (New York: Norton, 2006), p. 684/808.
14  Lacan, Jacques, "Position of the Unconscious," in *Écrits* (New York: Norton, 2006), p. 712/839–840 [translation modified].
15  Cf., for instance, Freud's, Sigmund, "Sexuality in the Etiology of Neurosis" (1898), in *Standard Edition*, Vol.III.; "Fragments of the Analysis of a Case of Hysteria" (1905), in *Standard Edition*, Vol.VII; "Analysis of a Phobia in Five-Year-Old Boy" (1909), in *Standard Edition*, Vol.X; "Totem and Taboo" (1912–1913), in *Standard Edition*, Vol.XIII; and "From the History of an Infantile Neurosis" (1918), in *Standard Edition*, Vol.XVII.
16  Lacan, Jacques, "The Function and Field of Speech in and Language in Psychoanalysis," in *Écrits* (New York: Norton, 2006), p. 213/256.
17  Cf. Hawking, Stephen & Mlodinow, Leopold, *The Grand Design* (New York: Random House, 2010), p. 72.
18  Lacan, Jacques, "Position of the Unconscious," in *Écrits* (New York: Norton, 2006), p. 711/839.
19  Lacan, Jacques, "Position of the Unconscious," in *Écrits* (New York: Norton, 2006), p. 713/841.
20  Lacan, Jacques, *Seminar XI*, p. 269.
21  Lacan, Jacques, "Position of the Unconscious…," in *Écrits* (New York: Norton, 2006), and *Seminar XI*, sessions XVI and XVII.
22  Eidelsztein, Alfredo, *Las estructuras clínicas a partir de Lacan*, vol.1 (Buenos Aires: Letra Viva, 2008), p. 43 ff.
23  Lacan, Jacques, "Position of the Unconscious…," in *Écrits* (New York: Norton, 2006), p. 716/844.
24  Eidelzstein, Alfredo, *The Graph of Desire. Using the Work of Jacques Lacan* (London: Karnac, 2009).
25  Lacan, Jacques, *Seminar IX*, session of 05.23.1962 [*Staferla*, p. 458].
26  Eidelsztein, Alfredo, "Lo simbólico en la obra de Jacques Lacan," in *El rey está desnudo*, Año 3, No.4 (2011).
27  The function of the hole is already present in Lacan's teaching before his encounter with the Borromean knot.
28  Lacan, Jacques, *Seminar XII*, session of 01.13.1965 [*Staferla*, p. 129].
29  Derrida, Jacques, "Structure, Sign, and Play in the Discourse of the Human Sciences," in *Writing and Difference* (London and New York: Routledge and Kegan Paul, 1978).
30  Kapuściński, Ryszard, *Travels with Herodotus* (New York: Knopf, 2008), p. 64.
31  However, sometimes, Lacan himself uses the expressions "speaking being" and "speaking animal."
32  Lacan, Jacques, *Seminar XX*, p. 32.
33  Freud, Sigmund, "The Question of Lay Analysis" (1926), in the *Standard Edition*, Vol. 20, p. 188.
34  Lacan, Jacques, *Seminar II*, p. 291.
35  In their view, this singularity is what distinguishes psychoanalysis from the biological sciences. Certainly, many biologists share this view (cf., for instance, Dawking, Richard, *The Selfish Gene* [Oxford: Oxford University Press, 2016]).

36  Lacan Jacques, "Subversion of the Subject and the Dialectic of Desire in the Freudian Unconscious," in *Écrits* (New York: Norton, 2006), p. 694.

37  Reichenbach, Hans, *The Rise of Scientific Philosophy* (Berkeley, Los Angeles and London: University of California Press, 1951), p. 174.

38  Among many authors, Norbert Elias in his *The Society of Individuals* (New York and London: Continuum, 1991) and Alain de Libera in his *Archéologie du sujet, vol.1. Naissance du sujet* (Paris: Librairie Phylosophique J. Vrin, 2007), offer sufficient arguments to criticize such prejudice.

39  de Libera, Alain, *Archéologie du sujet, vol.1. Naissance du sujet* (Paris: Librairie Phylosophique J. Vrin, 2007), p. 35.

40  Eidelsztein, Alfredo, "La responsabilidad subjetiva," in *El Rey está desnudo*, Año 8, No.8, 2015.

41  Cf. Freud, Sigmund, "Moral Responsibility for the Content of Dreams," a section of "Some Additional Notes on Dream-Interpretation as a Whole" (1925), in the *Standard Edition*, Vol.XIX.

42  Lacan, Jacques, "Position of the Unconscious," in *Écrits* (New York: Norton, 2006), p. 708/835.

43  Lacan, Jacques, *Seminar XIII*, session of 03.23.66 [*Staferla*, p. 377].

44  Cf. Lacan, Jacques, "Response to Jean Hyppolite's Commentary on Freud's '*Vermeinung*,'" in *Écrits* (New York: Norton, 2006), pp. 318–333, pp. 328–329. Cf., also, Lacan's *Seminar XIII*, session of 03.23.1966 [*Staferla*, p. 375.] and *Seminar XVI*, class of 11.20.68 [*Staferla*, p. 16].

45  de Libera, Alain, *Archéologie du sujet, vol.1. Naissance du sujet* (Paris: Librairie Phylosophique J. Vrin, 2007), p. 100 ff.

46  Lacan, Jacques, *Seminar XVII*, p. 77.

47  See my "Brief Presentation of the Big Bang Theory" at the end of this book (pp. 69–71).

48  Hawking, Stephen, *A Brief History of Time. From the Big Bang to Black Holes* (New York: Random House, 2011), p. 49.

49  Bojowald, Martin, *Once Before Time. A Whole History of the Universe* (New York: Alfred A. Kopf, 2010), p. 158.

50  Bojowald, Martin, *Once Before Time. A Whole History of the Universe* (New York: Alfred A. Kopf, 2010), p. 125.

51  Bojowald, Martin, *Once Before Time. A Whole History of the Universe* (New York: Alfred A. Kopf, 2010), p. 235.

52  Bojowald, Martin, *Once Before Time. A Whole History of the Universe* (New York: Alfred A. Kopf, 2010), p. 235.

53  Hawking, Stephen & Mlodinow, Leonard, *The Grand Design* (New York: Random House, 2010), p. 51.

54  Gangui, Alejandro, *El big bang. La génesis de nuestra cosmología actual* (Buenos Aires: EUDEBA, 2010), p. 241.

55  This is how I propose to translate the title of Lacan's conference paper and writing. In "*Fonction et champ de la parole en psychanalyse*" [Function and Field of Speech in Psychoanalysis], "parole," even when it could adequately be rendered as "word" and "speech," should be translated, as suggested by the content of the text, as "speech-act."

56  It all seems to suggest that Lacan never articulated his own conceptions with the big bang theory. I think this is because he did not get to know the theory. Otherwise, he always kept psychoanalysis entirely articulated with those scientific developments of his time that were in correspondence with his theoretical model.

57  Lacan does not take into account scientific developments solely in virtue of their quality of being modern, but he articulates them with his theoretical model on the basis of their philosophical and epistemological accounts. Thus, for instance, he criticizes Einstein's rejection of the fundamental principles of quantum physics. Already in

*Seminar II* Lacan started to consider Einstein's rejection of the probabilistic structure of reality—at the same time that he examined the uncertainty principle proposed by W. Heisenberg—posited by quantum physics and the most subversive consequence of Einstein's physical theory. Indeed, Lacan proposed a revision of the claim that embodied Einstein's stance in his correspondence with M. Born: "God does not play dice" (Lacan quotes it in *Seminar XII*, 11th session and also in *Seminar II*, 18th session, *Seminar XI*, 10th session, and *Seminar XIII*, 9th session). This is the reason why Lacan accused Einstein of "some kind of obscurantism" (*Seminar XVI*, 18th session). However, he never ceased to acknowledge and elaborate on the achievements of Einstein and H. Poincaré's relativistic physics (*Seminar XVIII*, 7th session; *Radiophone*, 4th question, and *Seminar XXI*, 4.23.1974). As for Einstein's formulas, he always stressed their value in that they establish an equivalence between matter and energy (*Seminar III*, 14th session) and underlined their strict signifying nature.

58  Lacan, Jacques, "Position of the Unconscious," in *Écrits* (New York: Norton, 2006), p. 713/841 [translation modified].

59  Later in the book I list some of the empirical research conducted within the ever-growing biologistic paradigm, as reported daily by many articles published in mass media.

60  Anthropological research on the oldest inscriptions (30,000 years old) always reveals a system: even when consisting of a very basic set of traces, there is never a trace that could be considered to be the first one. Cf. Gimbutas, Marija, *The Language of the Goddess* (New York: Harper, 1991).

61  The author is referring to the hundreds of existing African languages [*TN*].

62  Kapuscinski, Ryszard, *Travels with Herodotus* ((New York: Knopf, 2008), p. 171.

63  Voltaire, "Dictionnaire philosophique," in Œuvres completes de Voltaire, First Section: Langues-Génie des langues. Online resource: www.voltaire-integral.com/19/langues.htm (last accessed: May 14, 2023).

64  *Unidos por la lengua. Juventud y madurez*, online resource: www.celtiberia.net (last accessed: May 14, 2023).

65  Hurtado González, Silvia, *Los periodistas y la lengua*. Online resource: www.ucm.es/info/periodI/Period_I (last accessed: May 14, 2023).

66  Robert, Paul, *Dictionnaire de la langue française. Le grand Robert*, volume 4 (Paris: Aubin Imprimeur, 1994), p. 877.

67  Vázquez-Ayora, Gerardo, *Introducción a la traductología* (Washington, DC: Georgetown University School of Languages and Linguistics, 1977), pp. 85–87.

68  Cf. Grijelmo, Alex, *La seducción de las palabras: un recorrido por las manipulaciones del pensamiento* (Madrid: Taurus, 2000).

69  Benveniste, Émile, *Problems in General Linguistics* (Miami: University of Miami Press, 1971), p. 58.

70  Benveniste, Émile, *Problems in General Linguistics* (Miami: University of Miami Press, 1971), p. 61.

71  Kemplerer, Viktor, *The Language of the Third Reich. LTI – Lingua Tertii Imperii. A Philologist's Notebook* (London and New York: Bloomsbury, 2013).

72  Barthes, Roland, "Lecture in Inauguration of the Chair of Literary Semiology," *Collège de France*, January 7, 1977, in *October*, Vol. 8 (Spring, 1979), pp. 3–16.

73  Lacan, Jacques, "On Psychic Causality," in *Écrits* (New York: Norton, 2006), p. 140/171.

74  Lacan, Jacques, *Seminar VI*, 05.20.1959, *Staferla*, p. 650.

75  Lacan, Jacques, *Seminar VII*, p. 275.

76  Lacan, Jacques, *Seminar IX*, 06.27.1962. *Staferla*, p. 589.

77  Lacan, Jacques, *Seminar XXI*, 04.23.1974, *Staferla*, p. 215.

78  Dodds, Eric Robertson, *The Greeks and the Irrational* (Berkeley and Los Angeles: University of California Press, 1951), section IV: "Dream-Pattern and Culture-Pattern."

79  Lacan, Jacques, *L'étourdit* [I quote from Anthony Chadwick's translation, available here: http://www.lacanianworks.net/?p=221, pp. 467–468; NT].

80  Lacan, Jacques, "The Instance of the Letter in the Unconscious or Reason since Freud," in *Écrits* (New York: Norton, 2006), p. 414/495.

81  Foucault, for instance, argues that sex is an idea: "Is 'sex' really the anchorage point that supports the manifestations of sexuality, or is it not rather a complex idea that was formed inside the deployment of sexuality? In any case, one could show how this idea of sex took form in the different strategies of power and the definite role it played therein." Cf. Foucault, Michel, *History of Sexuality I. The Will to Power* (New York: Pantheon Book, 1978), p. 152.

82  Lacan, Jacques, *Seminar XX*, p. 33.

83  Lacan, Jacques, "Subversion of the Unconscious…," in *Écrits* (New York: Norton, 2006), p. 680/804. Lacan obtains the core argument of this famous passage from Herodotus' *The Nine Books of History*. I owe this reference to Federico Ludueña.

84  Bordelois, Yvonne, *Etimología de las pasiones* (Buenos Aires: Libros del Zorzal, 2006).

85  Morris, David, *The Culture of Pain* (Berkeley, Los Angeles and London: University of California Press, 1991), p. 20.

86  Morris, David, *The Culture of Pain* (Berkeley, Los Angeles and London: University of California Press, 1991), p. 5. By examining very serious research on the topic, the author argues that pain can be thought of as being culturally constructed.

87  Morris, David, *The Culture of Pain* (Berkeley, Los Angeles and London: University of California Press, 1991), p. 25.

88  Fischer, Seymour & Greenberg, Roger P., *The Limits of Biological Treatments for Psychological Distress-Comparisons with Psychotherapy and Placebo* (New York: Routledge, 2016), p. XIV.

89  Both *Clarín* and *La Nación* are Argentinean newspapers of widespread circulation [TN].

90  Sadly, as it has been noticed by many of the scholars working on these issues, in Western modern languages this is a difference—one that the Greeks named with the terms *bíos* and *zoe* (G. Agamben makes interesting remarks about it)—that was lost. *Bíos* indicates the *parlêtre*'s "life;" *zoe* refers to animal life. Today, particularly in the laboratories where medical and psychological research are conducted, these two meanings are mixed.

91  Lacan, Jacques, *Écrits* (New York: Norton, 2006), p. 145/178.

92  Wilson, Edmund O., *Sociobiology. The New Synthesis* (Cambridge, MA, and London: Belknap Press, 1975), p. 4.

93  Dawkins, Richard, *The Selfish Gene* (Oxford: Oxford University Press, 2016), p. 13.

94  Pinker, Steven, *The Language Instinct. How the Mind Creates Language* (New York: W. Morrow & Co., 1994), p. 362ff.

95  Pinker, Steven, *The Instinct of Language The Language Instinct. How the Mind Creates Language* (New York: W. Morrow & Co., 1994), p. 409.

96  Pinker, Steven, *The Language Instinct. How the Mind Creates Language* (New York: W. Morrow & Co., 1994), p. 365.

97  In this chapter, Pinker criticizes Elizabeth Bates, well-known for rejecting Chomsky's notion of a Universal Grammar and claiming that the latter must have appeared either as given by the Creator or as a big bang; further, Bates argues that the notion must be completely and utterly rejected. As she defends a constructivist logic of language, she rejects a big bang of language, for this idea entails a discontinuity. Pinker, by arguing for an instinct of language, must admit its sudden emergence.

98  Pinker, Steven, *The Language Instinct. How the Mind Creates Language* (New York: W. Morrow & Co., 1994), p. 342.

 99 Pinker, Steven, *The Language Instinct. How the Mind Creates Language* (New York: W. Morrow & Co., 1994), p. 351.

100 Pinker, Steven, *The Language Instinct. How the Mind Creates Language* (New York: W. Morrow & Co., 1994), p. 366.

101 See www.pinker.ejh.harvard.edu/about (last accessed: May 17, 2023).

102 According to Michel Foucault, the political honor of psychoanalysis lies in opposing the system of the symbolic order's law to the rampant ascent of contemporary racism (the man of flesh) [Foucault, Michel, *History of Sexuality. Volume 1: The Will to Power* (New York: Pantheon Book, 1978), p. 150]. It should be noted, though, that psychoanalysis can only accomplish such a project only if the analyst's position is conducive to that aim: if (s)he is rooted in the notion that the drives and *jouissance* are originated in the flesh, then (s)he will remain part of the racist movement, one that remains extremely pervasive in our time and culture.

103 Lacan, Jacques, *Seminar XXIII*, session of 11.18.75 [*Staferla*, p. 6] [Translation modified; TN].

104 Lacan, Jacques, "L'étourdit," in *Autres Écrits* (New York: Norton, 2006), p. 449.

105 Einstein, Albert & Infeld, Leopold, *The Evolution of Physics* (New York: Simon & Schuster, 1966), p. 244.

106 Freud, Sigmund, "The Metamorphosis of Puberty. 3. The Theory of Libido," in the *Standard Edition*, Vol.VII.

107 Lacan, Jacques, *Escritos 2, Position of the Unconscious, Seminar XI* (15th and 16th sessions) and *Seminar XXIII* (2nd session).

108 Hawking, Stephen & Mlodinov, Leonard, *The Grand Design* (New York: Random House, 2010), p. 82.

109 Rosenblum, Bruce & Kuttner, Fred, *Quantum Enigma. Physical Encounters with Consciousness* (New York: Oxford University Press, 2010), p. 4.

110 Lacan, Jacques, *Seminar II*, p. 240.

111 I would not claim the same regarding the usage of chemical formulae or the human genome, as I obviously accept that, in its own operative level and due to their formalization, the terms or concepts used in these disciplines do not function as terms of a natural language.

112 H. Casimir relates that the quantum physicists Bohr and Heisenberg once had a discussion on the nature of ontology at the house of the philosopher Hoffding; at some point in the conversation, Bohr claimed, "To be…to be…what does it *mean* to be?" (Quoted by Amir Axel in his book, *Entanglement. The Greatest Mystery in Physics* [New York: Four Walls Eight Windows, 2002], p. 88).

113 Badiou, Alain, *Being and Event* (New York: Bloomsbury, 2013) and Meillassoux, Quentin, *After Finitude. Essay on the Necessity of Contingency* (Paris: du Seuil, 2006). Both philosophical works are built on mathematical foundations.

114 Einstein, Albert & Infeld, Leopold, *The Evolution of Physics* (New York: Simon & Schuster, 1966), p. 129.

115 Gangui, Alejandro, *El big bang. La génesis de nuestra cosmología actual* (Buenos Aires: EUDEBA, 2010), p. 132.

116 For modern physics, the definition of the void is: the state that has the least possible energy. Cf. Peter, Patrick and Gangui, Alejandro, *Des défauts dans l'Univers* (Paris: CNRS, 2003).

117 Cf. Rosenblum, Bruce & Kuttner, Fred, *Quantum Enigma. Physical Encounters with Consciousness* (New York: Oxford University Press, 2010).

118 Lacan, *Seminar XVII*, session of 03.11.1970 [*Staferla*, pp. 146–147; my translation is from the French and Eidelsztein's own translation to Spanish; I have also consulted Cormac Gallagher's unpublished translation of Lacan's seminar {TN}].

119 Cf. Lacan, Jacques, *Escritos 1. Intervención sobre la transferencia* (2008), p. 210.

120 Pommier, Gérard, *Cómo las neurociencias demuestran el psicoanálisis* (Buenos Aires: Letra Viva, 2010). Pommier's book was recommended as a "friendly book" by Phoenix S.A.I.C. and F., a laboratory of medical products, a few months after its publication.

121 Miller, Jacques-Alain, *El Otro que no existe y sus comités de ética* (Barcelona and México: Paidós, 2005), pp. 193, 383, and 416.

122 Lacan, Jacques, *Seminar XXIII*, session of 01.13.76 [Staferla, p. 37]. Cf, also, *Psicoanálisis. Radiofonía y Televisión* (Buenos Aires: Anagrama, 1977), pp. 86–94.

123 Lacan, Jacques, "Position of the Unconscious," in *Écrits* (New York: Norton, 2006), p. 715/843.

124 Lacan, Jacques, "Of Structure as an Inmixing of an Otherness Prerequisite to Any Subject Whatever," in Macksey, Richard & Donato, Eugenio (eds.), *The Structuralist Controversy. The Languages of Criticism and the Sciences of Man* (Baltimore, MD and London: The John Hopkins University Press, 1979). 10.21.1966. Online resource: https://www.lacan.com/hotel.htm (last accessed: July 4, 2021). Lacan's presentation was published in *The Languages of Criticism and the Sciences of Man: The Structuralist Controversy*, R. Macksey and E. Donato (eds.) (Baltimore, MD: Johns Hopkins Press, 1970).

125 Durkheim, Émile, *The Elementary Forms of Religious Life* (Oxford: Oxford University Press, 2001), p. 199.

126 With Lacan, I make a distinction between sense and meaning. The former unequivocally refers to the signifying universe: it is entirely absent in the animal world. Further, it indicates the problematic stance of the Other (A) in all saying. Lacan puts it as follows: "This is what you tell me, but, what do you want?" Sense, so construed, coincides with the specific function of the question and goes beyond any given text. The realization of sense does not coincide with the vanishing of this aspect of the question, but with the falling into non-sense.

127 Eidelsztein, Alfredo, *Las estructuras clínicas a partir de Lacan*, vol.1 (Buenos Aires: Letra Viva, 2008).

128 *Pas-tout-Lacan*, Available on: www.ecolelacanienne.net, p. 1438 (last accessed: July 10, 2021).

129 Balivar, François, *Histoires des sciences. Einstein et Poincaré, une affaire des principes* (Paris: Belin, 2008).

130 For an accessible presentation of this theory, see Greene, Brian, *The Fabric of the Cosmos. Space, Time, and the Texture of Reality* (New York: Alfred Knopf, 2004).

131 Bojowald, Martin, *Once Before Time. A Whole History of the Universe* (New York: Alfred A. Kopf, 2010), p. 80.

132 Bojowald, Martin, *Once Before Time. A Whole History of the Universe* (New York: Alfred A. Kopf, 2010), p. 44.

133 Cf. Einstein, Albert and Infeld, Leopold, *The Evolution of Physics* (New York: Simon & Schuster, 1966), p. 217.

134 Einstein, Albert and Infeld, Leopold, *The Evolution of Physics* (New York: Simon & Schuster, 1966), p. 221

135 Reichenbach, Hans, *The Rise of Scientific Philosophy* (Berkeley, Los Angeles and London: University of California Press, 1951), p. 183.

136 Einstein, Albert & Infeld, Leopold, *The Evolution of Physics* (New York: Simon & Schuster, 1966), pp. 157–158.

137 Einstein, Albert & Infeld, Leopold, *The Evolution of Physics* (New York: Simon & Schuster, 1966), pp. 258–259.

138 Reichenbach, Hans, *The Rise of Scientific Philosophy* (Berkeley, Los Angeles and London: University of California Press, 1951), p. 189.

139 Hawking, Stephen & Mlodinow, Leopold, *The Grand Design* (New York: Random House, 2010), p. 67.

140  Lacan, Jacques, *Seminar XVII*, p. 159.
141  Lacan, Jacques, "Geneva Conference on the Symptom," in *Analysis*, No.1, 1989, pp. 7–26. (The text can be found here: https://freud2lacan.b-cdn.net/Geneva_Lecture. pdf; TN.)
142  Elias, Norbert, *The Society of Individuals* (New York and London: Continuum, 1991), pp. 31–32.
143  Einstein, Albert & Infeld, Leopold, *The Evolution of Physics* (New York: Simon & Schuster, 1966), p. 152.
144  Lovejoy, Arthur O., *The Great Chain of Being. History on an Idea.*
145  Sala Rose, Rosa., *Diccionario crítico de mitos y símbolos del nazismo* (Barcelona: El Acantilado,2003).
146  Wilson, Edmund O., *Sociobiology. The New Synthesis* (Cambridge, MA, and London: Belknap Press, 1975).
147  Damasio, Antonio, *Descartes' Error. Emotion, Reason, and the Human Brain* (New York: Penguin, 2005).
148  Ambrogi, Adelaide (ed.), *Filosofía de la ciencia. El giro naturalista* (Barcelona: Ediciones de la UIB, 1999).
149  Gould, Stephen J., *Ontogeny and Phylogeny* (Cambridge, MA: Belknap Press, 1977).
150  Freud, Sigmund, "Moses and Monotheism," in Freud, *SE*, vol.XXIII.
151  Miller, Jacques-Alain, "Lacanian Biology and the Event of the Body," in *The Symptom*, 18 (available on-line here: https://www.lacan.com/symptom/lacanian-biology-miller/ (part I) and here: https://www.lacan.com/symptom/lacanian-biology-and-the-event-of-the-body-part-ii/ (part II); last accessed: May 14, 2023; NT).
152  Levi-Strauss, Claude, *Race and History* (Ann Arbor: University of Michigan Press, 1961).

# Chapter 4

# The Symbolic in Lacan, or the Function of the Hole

As Lacan maintained a few months before his death in the seminar he gave in Caracas, the three registers he proposed for psychoanalysis constitute a paradigm destined to *replace* the second topography bequeathed by Freud to his disciples. It is a paradigm that entails a radically new structure in terms of its elements as well as its laws of composition. This is a novelty with respect to what Freud proposed, but also with respect to what the common sense of our time and society designates: the Imaginary, the Symbolic, and the Real.

From a social and cultural perspective, the Imaginary tends to be presented as what we imagine: a world of fantasy, which operates like a crystal each of us carries, knowingly or not, through which the world is colored in an individual and unique way. The Symbolic is usually conceived as a package of positive symbols, conventional signs through which we represent reality, its objects, and its phenomena. Finally, the Real is typically thought of as a material substance, posited either as "flesh," i.e., the "internal" material constitutive of each individual, or as "stone," i.e., the objective "exterior" that surrounds each person. It is also generally claimed that the Imaginary veils the Real and that the Symbolic cannot fully represent it.

With respect to Freud's second paradigm—that of the ego, superego, *id*, and reality—Lacan's position could hardly be more different, despite his disciples' attempts to show not only that there is no discontinuity between them, but also that they are almost identical, as if Lacan's position were only a transcription, with new names, of the old Freudian elements.

Far from it, in this conceptual field the differences between Freud and Lacan are radical. Take, for instance, their concepts of ego. For Freud, the ego is internal and central, loved by us. As the object of our love, the ego functions as the narcissistic basis for all object-love. It is also the most faithful witness of reality, since, in Freud's conception, it consists of the mnemic traces of experiences of satisfaction that occur at the beginning of life. Finally, the ego is the foundational basis of our internal world (the "real" world, in his view, is the "outside" where all unsatisfactory experiences are deposited). For Lacan, the ego is the exact opposite, namely, the inevitable confusion between ego and other, which Lacan writes in his algebraic aa'. Further, this confusion produces the paradoxical "I am other," the basis of alienation, which establishes not love but the characteristic aggressiveness of the ego.

DOI: 10.4324/9781003485339-6

Another unnoticed, silenced difference between their conceptions is the following: for Freud, the *id* is the source of the drives that originate within the biological body and affect the psychic apparatus, whereas for Lacan, it works according to an entirely different logic. His conceptualization of the *ça* indicates that *ça pense* and *ça parle*[1] are *impersonal* processes of thought and speech that cannot be understood through an individualistic framework.[2] Thus, Freud's and Lacan's views clearly contradict each other.

Yet another difference between Freud and Lacan is that the former developed two distinct paradigms, known as the first and second topographies, whereas Lacan consistently defended the same one, from the beginning of his teaching in 1953 to his death. This is true despite his followers' efforts to differentiate a first, second, and third stage in Lacan's teaching, as if he could be read in evolutionary terms.

Let us now examine in detail the structure of the Symbolic, the Imaginary, and the Real in the Borromean knot (see figure below) as Lacan formulated it from the 1970s onwards. In this structure, the Imaginary ring goes over the Real, and the Real goes over the Symbolic, which, in turn, goes over the Imaginary. Thus, their relation can be described as the links of a chain where each link is interpenetrated by the other two.

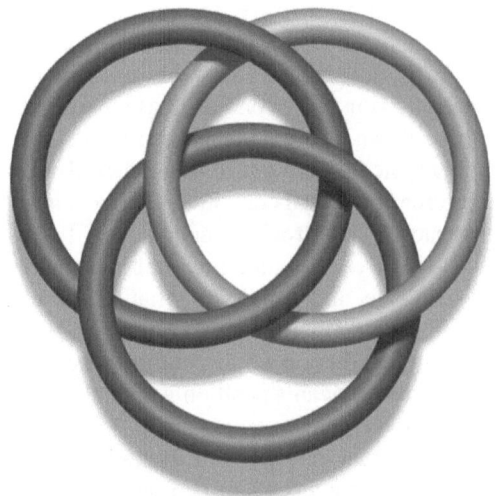

The logic that accounts for the proper and specific relation among the Symbolic, the Imaginary, and the Real is that of the Borromean knot. Here, Lacan's insight advances a substantial novelty: each of the three elements exists only in the tripartite relationship with the other two, and this is the sole way that they can be articulated. This point should be heavily stressed: they can *only* be in relation to each other. It is thus clear that, for Lacan, being is rooted and consists only in a relation, which must be understood radically as follows: being *itself* is relational.

In particular, no *parlêtre* exists alone, i.e., as separate from the relationships that constitute it, so both the *parlêtre* itself and its relationships with other *parlêtres* are thought of as "links" or "loops." Psychoanalysis itself is conceived by Lacan as a discourse and, consequently, as a social *link*, so much so that Lacan, stressing the value of the link, i.e., the fundamental importance of the articulation of the elements of discourse, is able to claim that "there is no such thing as prediscursive reality."[3]

Other authors in the social sciences make similar proposals, but they are lesser-known. Norbert Elias, for instance, argues in his historical sociology that man's being must be thought of in relational (not individualistic) terms, stressing that the West is governed by the prejudice that the individual is real and that relations are thought of as ideal presuppositions.[4] In his view, the human world is characterized by its "entanglement," which surprisingly coincides with what is now called by physicists the "greatest mystery of quantum physics:" the entangled existence of subatomic particles.[5]

Strictly speaking, the being of the chain with which Lacan operates is to be found exclusively in the relationship between the links of the chain, so their material (rope, iron, etc.) only constitutes an anchor for imagination. For Lacan links are in fact toric surfaces and, as such, two-dimensional and intangible topological surfaces.

In Freud's system each element is in itself independent from, though it must bear the incidences of, all others, which, naturally, is also applicable to the ego (the vassal of the superego), the *id*, and reality. This is also how, for Freud, the individual functions in society. For Lacan, however, *every* entity or element in psychoanalysis (especially the subject) must be taken as a signifier, i.e., as an element whose being *is* in relation to what it *is not*.

At the heart of Lacan's theory lies his theory of the signifier. The whole of his philosophical enterprise, his *matérialisme* (a materialism of the word, of speech),[6] entails the positing of a series of fundamental ideas: (1) the *parlêtre* (a "speaking-being" or, better, a "being-spoken," where its being is inseparable from the phenomenon of language, of which it is a manifestation),[7] (2) *hontologie* (indicating that the thesis "being is and non-being is not" is a shameful [Fr. *honte*, Eng. *shame*] ontological claim),[8] and (3) unsubstance (expressing his rejection of our prevailing reifying and objectifying [*cosificadora*] ideology).[9] Thus, Lacan's is a true anti-philosophy, one that rests entirely on his theory of the signifier.[10]

In Lacan's account signifiers only exist in the element of language and in their difference from all other signifiers. Further, they consist in the empty place left by all others, and, in analytic practice, they occupy a position relative to other signifiers in the signifying chain. In Lacan's own terms: "... there are in this world signifiers that mean nothing and must be deciphered ...".[11]

From the very beginning of his elaboration of the Symbolic, Lacan thinks of it as the register that ties the other two together, since it provides the function of the knot. This happens through the signifying operation: each signifier exists in at least a dual relation, which can be posited as that of $S_1$ and $S_2$ (see figure below), that serves as the foundation for a reversible time and a circular combinatorial space, both constituted by the signifying relation in the form of a loop or closed line.[12] In the signifying chain, the first signifier anticipates the second, and the latter resignifies the first.

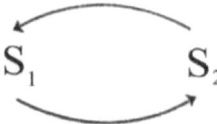

Through the notion of loop or closed lined, Lacan conceptualized first, the signifying interval, then the signifier's circular trajectory, and finally the signifier's creation of the hole, the main topic of this chapter, which I now address in some detail.

From the moment Lacan was able to conceive of topology as the necessary space for psychoanalysis (*Seminar IX* on identification), he maintains the following argument—one he would never abandon: "This line that we call 'the cut' is a line— this is our starting point—that we must conceive aprioristically as closed. It is the signifier's essence."[13]

The closed line, the signifying loop, captures the essence of what Lacan previously indicated as the signifying interval. It is a two-dimensional place where the subject (posited as what one signifier represents to another signifier, a formula produced precisely in these same years), the Other (which cannot be completed through a meta-language), and the acosmic *object a* exist.

These theoretical findings consolidate the development of the logic of the hole and give it its proper place and full value in Lacan's psychoanalysis. The hole provides the logical possibility of *béance*.[14] This term comes from the French word *béer*—desire—and means both a state of being open as well as an opening. In English, it could be translated as "hollowness" (Fr. *ouverture*).

The hole operates as a whirlpool, as a "devouring cyclone," which, in the *parlêtre's* universe, absorbs and annihilates material substance as the cause of desire's movement, creating thereby the *object a*.

In topology, the hole, contrary to the presupposition that legitimizes Freud's notion of castration, in no way indicates something missing, or something that has been removed, rather, it is a fundamental property of the structure.[15]

The problem at stake in the opposition between the prevailing ideology and Lacan's theory can be clearly observed in the usual identification of "circle"—a full surface without a hole—with "circumference"—a closed line dividing a surface in two. We often speak of a circle when in fact we mean to refer to a circumference. Our inclination, then, is to "fill" and "plug" what seems to circumscribe a hole.

It is in virtue of the fundamental value of the hole that Lacan claims that his topology is a geometry that repudiates its name.[16] Indeed, topology operates exclusively with surfaces capable of accommodating holes, from which one should not draw the conclusion that it can accommodate solids, as the earth in "geometry."

For Lacan's psychoanalysis, the hole is created by the signifier, so the Symbolic is specified as "… the dimension of the signifier that creates a hole …".[17] Thus, Lacan's Symbolic has a circular trajectory and consists only in the hole created by it.[18]

For Lacan, Freud's concept of the unconscious implies only one thing, namely, the positing of a *fiat* hole, equivalent to the *fiat lux*[19] of the Judeo-Christian tradition.[20] The Freudian thing, for Lacan, dwells solely in the hole that exists in the Symbolic.

Finally, let us briefly examine Lacan's most elaborated psychoanalytic account of the hole, the Borromean knot:

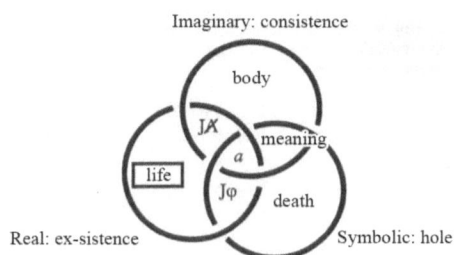

Notice that the Symbolic is characterized by the hole, not by the symbol; the Imaginary, by bodily consistency, not by phantasies or images, imagined or otherwise; and the Real, by ex-istences, not by three-dimensional entities. The three registers exist only in their reciprocal relation, as knotted, each one chained to the other two. This is made possible by the Symbolic of the hole, caused in turn by the operation of the signifier.

It may be said that, on the one hand, the Symbolic provides the hole, which is the condition for the interlacing of the rings; on the other hand, that the Symbolic exists only as knotted to the other two registers, which indicates the logical necessity of reversible time. These apparently contradictory theses are simultaneously true.

Indeed, (a) the Symbolic is the hole. (b) The Imaginary is everything that, having a three-dimensional consistency, plugs the hole. This consistency is not logical, and its aim is to obliterate or obstruct the hole. In our epoch and society, consistency is eminently conceived as the body as flesh. (c) Contrary to what is taken for granted among Freudo-Lacanian psychoanalysts, the Real is neither the bone nor the stone, but the ex-istence, i.e., the life, of beings such as God, the unconscious, and logico-mathematical impossibilities, which ex-ist and are created in the possibility opened up by the symbolic hole.

Even *jouissance*, one of Lacan's most creative concepts, is predominantly understood in such a way that the novelty of Lacan's notion of the hole is erased. It is, in fact, typically equated with unsatisfactory satisfaction and pleasurable displeasure thought to originate in biological substance. Quite the opposite. For Lacan, as we read in his Borromean knot, *jouissance* is also inscribed in the holes, which should not be confused with Freud's erogenous zones. For Freud, the latter are those areas of the living being's integument strongly innervated by nerve endings. For Lacan, on the other hand, the signifying hole, functioning like a cyclone, devours such zones from our lives. For Freud, the bodily holes are inside the edge of the skin or mucosa, whereas, for Lacan, the holes are both "in" and "out" the biological *soma*, thus creating a new logic—that of the "extimacy" (*extimité*).

## Notes

1  See *Ça parle (it speaks), ça pense (it thinks), and Subjective Responsibility*, in this volume, p. xxx.
2  Cf. Sarraillet, María Inés, "El sujeto del inconsciente como impersonal y el problema de la responsabilidad subjetiva," in *El Rey está desnudo*, 1 (Buenos Aires: Letra Viva, 2008), pp. 17–32.
3  Lacan, Jacques, *Seminar XX* (New York: Norton, 1998), p. 22.
4  Cf. Elias, Norbert, *The Society of Individuals* (New York and London: Continuum, 1991).
5  Cf. Aczel, Amir D., *Entanglement. The Greatest Mystery in Physics* (New York: Four Walls Eight Windows, 2002).
6  Lacan, Jacques, "Geneva Conference on the Symptom," in *Analysis*, 1:7 (Carlton South: Australian Center for Psychoanalysis, 1989), p. 14.
7  Lacan, Jacques, *La troisième. Staferla*.
8  Lacan, Jacques, *Seminar XVII* (New York: Norton, 2007), p. 195.
9  Lacan, Jacques, *Seminar XVII* (New York: Norton, 2007), p. 160.
10  Lacan, Jacques, "Peut-être à Vicennes" in *Autres écrits* (Paris: du Seuil. p. 314).
11  Lacan, Jacques, "Position of the Unconscious…" in Écrits (New York: Norton, 2006), p. 712/840.
12  In topology, a loop is technically a "closed Jordan curve."
13  Lacan, Jacques, *Seminar IX*. Session of 05.23.1962. Staferla, p. 161.
14  Lacan, Jacques, *Seminar IX*. Session of 05.23.1962. Staferla, p. 161.
15  Cf. Ruiz, C. Conferencia dentro del Ciclo Conferencias Clínicas Hospital Alvear. Octubre 2002.
16  Lacan, Jacques, *Seminar XXII*. Session of 04.15.1975. Staferla.
17  Lacan, Jacques, *Seminar XXII*. Session of 04.15.1975. Staferla.
18  Lacan, Jacques, *Journées des cartels de l'École freudienne de Paris. Maison de la chimie* (Paris: Lettre de l'École freudienne, 1976), n° 18, pp. 263–270, in *Pas-tout Lacan*, pp. 1701–1708.
19  "Let There Be Light."
20  Lacan, Jacques, *Journées des cartels de l'École freudienne de Paris. Maison de la chimie* (Paris: Lettre de l'École freudienne, 1976), n° 18, pp. 263–270.

# Chapter 5

# Logic and Psychoanalysis. Alienation, Separation, and the Ω Operation

The post-Freudian psychoanalysts (up to Lacan) forgot many of Freud's teachings and offered a considerable number of contributions to the psychoanalysis he invented. However, most of these additions entailed, in fact, nothing more than a return to a state of affairs that one may resolutely label "pre-Freudian." Among the most prominent of such oversights is that of the essentially logical status of the unconscious. For Freud, without a doubt, the most intimate and essential structure of the unconscious is logical in nature, and therefore, analytic work, both in theory and in practice, requires that this logic be elaborated. Further, the practice of psychoanalysis requires the establishment and formalization of a logic. Only Lacan, in his *Seminar IV* on the object relation, highlights this with total clarity:

> Freud already began in *The Interpretation of Dreams* to tell us something about the logic of the unconscious, in other words, about the signifiers in the unconscious. A whole quarter of *The Interpretation of Dreams* is devoted to showing how a certain number of essential logical articulations, the either-or, contradiction, causality, can be transposed into the order of the unconscious. This logic may be distinct from our customary logic. Just as topology is a geometry of rubber, here too it is a question of a logic in rubber.[1]

Given this degree of forgetfulness, or repression, it may be useful to recall what Freud claimed in some key passages of his work. In my view, though, the logic of the unconscious was developed not by Freud, but by Lacan. Indeed, if one revisits at least the following texts (there are many others), one will find both the origins as well as the foundations of this logic, but not its actual development: "Project for a Scientific Psychology;"[2] "The Psychotherapy of Hysteria;"[3] "The Interpretation of Dreams"[4] (especially "The Means of Representation in Dreams"); "On Dreams;"[5] "The Antithetical Meaning of Primal Words;"[6] "The Claims of Psychoanalysis to Scientific Interest;"[7] and the 11th introductory lecture, entitled "The Dream-Work."[8]

DOI: 10.4324/9781003485339-7

The logico-formal structure of Freud's unconscious can be summarized in the following famous passage from his "On the Psychotherapy of Hysteria" (as it is quite long, here is an abbreviated version):

> The psychical material [...] presents itself as a structure in several dimensions which is stratified in at least three different ways. [...] In the first place there is an unmistakable linear chronological order which obtains within each separate theme. [...] Each of them is—I cannot express it in any other way—stratified concentrically round the pathogenic nucleus. [...] A third kind of arrangement has still to be mentioned—the most important, but the one about which it is least easy to make any general statement. What I have in mind is an arrangement according to thought-content, the linkage made by a logical thread which reaches as far as the nucleus [...] This arrangement has a dynamic character, in contrast to the morphological one of the two stratifications mentioned previously. [...] Advances are brought about, as we know, by overcoming resistance in the manner already indicated. But before this, we have as a rule another task to perform. We must get hold of a piece of the logical thread, by whose guidance alone we may hope to penetrate to the interior.[9]

Among psychoanalysts, chronological ordering has always been emphasized, since in our culture historical evolution and linear progress are always preferred. Our conception of order in the style of cataphiles illustrates the same point, as it expresses that one always wants to assume a central core, a real trauma. Our culture works with the notion that there is a center and that this place is occupied by something (such as an internal bone or an external stone). In this way, we try to avoid confronting that lack is *structurally* necessary: lack of origin, lack of center, and lack of destination.[10] As a consequence, the most essential articulation, the logical one, has been forgotten. It is only through Lacan's teaching that it is possible to recuperate this dimension—the logical dimension of lack—and delve deeper into it. In his own words: the unconscious must be questioned until it gives an answer that does not take the form of a rapture or a demolition, but rather asks "why?"

> If we conduct the subject anywhere, it is to a deciphering which assumes that a sort of logic is already operative in the unconscious, a logic in which, for example, an interrogative voice or even the development of an argument can be recognized.[11]

It is clear that in this case Lacan is referring to the psychoanalytic clinic and to logical argumentation. For him, the decisive formulas of his conception of the unconscious are *logical* formulas, the same kind with which modern symbolic logic operates.[12]

Freud proposed that for his concept of the unconscious it was essential to question classical logic, since some of its principles were not applicable to his amazing discovery. Lacan, the only one who pursued this path, developed a specific logic for the subject of the unconscious through the operations of alienation and separation. He further elaborated on this logic by introducing the truth table he designated as "Ω" (omega).

## Alienation and Separation

For Lacan, alienation and separation are logical operations and not evolutionary moments, developmental periods, or stages of constitution. He makes it abundantly clear: it is a question of symbolic logic and mathematical set theory. Both in his seminars (especially those taught between 1964 and 1967, i.e., seminars XI to XIV) and in the chapter Position of the Unconscious," he demonstrates it with total clarity. Let us examine it in some depth.

Alienation is one of the operations that accounts for the relationship between subject (S) and Other (A)—with A referring to the structure of language—a relationship that Lacan describes as a "(…) fundamental and new logical opera-tion."[13] For Lacan, alienation has the same logical structure as a vel ("or"), but is alienating in nature. This vel, necessary for the logical conception of the sub-ject, has the structure of the "union" in mathematical set theory. It implies a loss of being as an effect of the structure of the signifying chain, which constitutes the "lethal factor" of the signifier.[14] Thus, alienation implies "neither one nor the other," which follows from the fact that the subject occupies a place always in-between the signifiers. Lacan had already developed these psychoanalytic principles when he elaborated his theory of the lack-in-being [*manque-à-être*] as an effect of metonymy.[15]

Separation, on the contrary, has the structure of the intersection in set theory. In its most radical dimension, it entails the set-up of what is lost in the advent of the subject.[16] It implies that what rescues the subject—not the person—from the lethal factor of the signifying pair is the encounter and articulation with the Other's lack (where "Other" means the embodiment of A). This is quite different from the crude metaphor of a subject being born out of itself, which would reintroduce the idea of individual liberation (exemplified in the self-made man). Following Lacan, what is lost in the advent of the subject may be called "libido," but this notion no longer refers to intrapsychic energy. What is lost, becoming, or functioning as, the *object a*, is the logical articulation, in desire and the drives, of the Other and its lack. Such desire will remain structurally unconscious and the drive will always be only a partial drive. The myth of the lamella, developed by Lacan in *Seminar XI*, comes to represent this dialectic, but it is a myth that does not offer any account of cause or origin. It is a partial dialectic, a dialectic of a part (*pars*) that is not a component of any whole.[17]

At this point in my argument, it is convenient to introduce a comment on a very frequent misreading of Lacan's notions of alienation and separation. It is my impression that many psychoanalysts consider alienation as dependence on the Other and separation as liberation and appropriation of one's own desire. There is no room for ambiguity here: for Lacan, the essential structure of man's desire is that of being the desire *of the Other*. One always desires the desire of the Other and there is no possibility that unconscious desire is expressed as "I desire x." All expressions such as "I desire" or "I desire x" are formulas offered by phantasy [*phantasme*] that function as a support for desire, but for Lacan there is no possibility of appropriating desire individually. No one can be the master of his desire, since "desire" and "master" are essentially contradictory terms. Lacan clearly emphasizes that freedom is a fantasy and that we must remember the alienation inherent in the position of the master.[18] The most radical way of rejecting desire is the wish to be rid of it. Thus, no one can take possession of his own desire. What makes possible the interpretation of desire is an act that posits the subject as invested by a particular desire that has at the same time the form of a "*one desires*" [*se desea*], a desire that always lies in the field of the Other, i.e., in the relation to the Other, the latter being the fundamental condition for the existence of a psychoanalytic subject.

It is through separation that Lacan conceives of the resolution of transference. This is another reason to distinguish alienation from any notion of dependence and also separation from freedom, so one avoids assuming, as all the detractors of psychoanalysis do (and, inadvertently, many analysts too), that (i) engaging in a psychoanalysis implies a loss of freedom (by alienating oneself to a new Other) and, therefore, dependence, and (ii) the operation of separation consists in separating oneself from the analyst, recovering thereby one's independence and autonomy. It can be argued that the relationship between the two logical operations is what makes it possible to account for the profound articulation, which is at the basis of transference, between the structure of the subject of the unconscious, the subject supposed to know, and (from Lacan's perspective) the logically necessary notion of the analyst's desire.

The only way to avoid transference becoming an effect of the Other's capacity for suggestion and its demand is to put to work in the analytic setting the function of the Other's desire represented as the analyst's desire—a desire which, beyond any demand, unconscious or not, characterizes analytic practice. Only in the analytic setting does the analyst's desire function as an *object a*, both as a cause of desire as well as the remnant of the analytic operation at the end of an analysis.

### The Ω Operation

Other than alienation and separation, Lacan identified as the ultimate feature of the unconscious' logic the truth table of the "Ω operation," which he also calls "the alienation operation."[19] This represents his attempt to provide a logical and formal foundation for his conception of the subject and the unconscious.

Notably forgotten and even unknown by his followers, this operation is characterized by a truth table that, deduced from the logic that governs the signifier in the unconscious, is described as "either I am not or I do not think," which indicates Lacan's transformation of the Cartesian cogito. It reads as follows:

| p | q | Ω |
|---|---|---|
| T | T | F |
| T | F | T |
| F | T | T |
| F | F | T |

As an F in the third column is only obtained when the truth values of the variables are both T, this table of truth-value is different from the canonical operations of symbolic logic:

| Conjunction | Inclusive Disjunction | Exclusive Disjunction | Implication | coimplication |
|---|---|---|---|---|
| "and" | "or" (vel) | "or" (aut) | "if..., then..." | "...if and only if..." |
| "∧" | "∨" | "∨" | "→" | "↔" |
| p q p ∧ q | p q p ∨ q | p q p ∨ q | p q p → q | p q p ↔ q |
| T T T | T T T | T T F | T T T | T T T |
| T F F | T F T | T F T | T F F | T F F |
| F T F | F T T | F T T | F T T | F T F |
| F F F | F F F | F F F | F F T | F F T |

Perhaps out of ignorance or a motive that escapes my analysis, nowhere in his teaching does Lacan clarify that the Ω truth table, rarely cited or used in standard logic textbooks, is known as symbolic logic as the truth table that corresponds to the Sheffer stroke (written "p | q").[20] The Sheffer stroke entails that "p and q are incompatible" (not true simultaneously) and that A | B <=> ¬ (A ∧ B).

It may be a mere coincidence, but it is noteworthy that the only example I have found of the logical use of incompatibility coincides strikingly with Lacan's account of alienation. It is the paradigm developed by R. Abarca, who argues that

> incompatibility means that the same person cannot be, at the same time, two different things; thus [for instance] it is incompatible to be a judge and a lawyer, as one person cannot act both as a judge and as a lawyer at the same time. Therefore, if the two atomic propositions were true, the molecular one would have to be false.[21]

In the table proposed by Lacan, the articulation of TT is false, whereas all the other combinations are true. This is equivalent to stating that: (a) contrary to the aforementioned example of the judge and the lawyer being incompatible, in the formula, "Either *I am not* or *I do not think*," one of the components must be false; (b) the ego does not operate in the unconscious, and (c) there is no true truth (TT).

This table is not usable in psychoanalysis as the others are used in symbolic logic. It clearly does not serve to establish whether a statement is true or false. Further, it does not allow us to interpret the truth at stake in the clinical material.

However, it does enable the logical presentation of a concept (the $\Omega$ operation) both in the analyst's training and in the presentation of cases in their clinical work.

In the same seminar where Lacan deals with the omega operation, a seminar almost entirely devoted to logic, he also presents other very significant articulations between psychoanalysis and symbolic logic. It is impossible to go through all of them here. I restrict myself to highlighting only the ones that provide a logical basis for the analysis of the Cartesian cogito in its relationship with the subject of science and with the unconscious, which psychoanalysis has been dealing with since Freud.

From all the developments made by Lacan in *Seminar XIV*, I would like to stress one more. It is his attempt to write the logic at play in an expression so often used by him: "not without," one that his followers tend to quote very frequently—as in the case of "anguish is not without an object"—while typically forgetting its logical basis. This logic is labeled by Lacan "not-without negation," by which he indicates that there are cases in which one must affirm that "this is not without that,"

> Now, there arises a form of negation that has nothing to do with the complementary negation of class logic and that we will call the not-without—this does not work without that—in order to underline the paradox that may emerge when one brings together two propositions by an implication (...).[22]

According to my reading of Lacan's text, the virtue of this maneuver consists in offering a version, in terms of symbolic logic, of the affirmation of the subject's lack-in-being (*manque-à-être*) in the unconscious that does not culminate in a nihilistic position (i.e., the pure lack of value, meaning, or truth). The lack-in-being does not operate without the *object a*.[23] Presence and absence, object and lack, creation ex-nihilo, and lack-in-being are intimately articulated in the logic of the subject proposed by Lacan.

In the rest of his teaching, Lacan continues the attempt to relate core psychoanalytic arguments and concepts with other logical and mathematical developments, such as: modal logic, his theorization of human sexuality in the formulas of sexuation through the use of logical quantifiers, and the Borromean knot as a way of articulating the three registers. However, even if one only takes into consideration the developments examined in this essay, he already counts with a minimal argumentative basis to offer a logical version of the subject of the unconscious, its relationship with the Other, the *object a*, desire, and the drives [*pulsión*]. To conclude, let me establish the consequences of the position of psychoanalysis regarding these logical issues.

From the establishment of the Cartesian cogito, subjectivity in the West has become intimately associated with knowledge as thought: I think, therefore I am. The modern subject thus characterized is the subject of science. Ever since, desire has been located between thought and knowledge. It is a desire that, according to Lacan, in our society and epoch, takes the form of a desire *to know*.[24] But if it is precisely a *desire* to know, there will necessarily be a dimension of nescience, i.e., of not-knowing, embedded in the field of knowledge, especially associated with the "I" (*je*) of the subject and with truth.

This unknown was designated by Freud as "the unconscious." Modern science tends to elaborate it in a reductionist manner. Psychoanalysis tries to reintroduce it into science and culture, not only as a generic "what is not known" by us, but as a particular "empty core" of not-knowing in each one of us, which operates as "an immixture of Otherness."[25] In our culture, a psychoanalytic position, regardless of its theoretical orientation, should entail the positing of a fundamental non-knowledge as a means to establish the subjective position of each one within the framework of the Other's field. My contention is that such a postulation should be studied, known, and formalized logically.

This mark introduced by psychoanalysis into culture is articulated to science because, from the first Freudian gesture, psychoanalysis was characterized by a style, a scientific way of sustaining its statements referring to the unknown and of creating a practice according to it in each particular case. Its clinic and its theory, if they can be said to exist separately, articulate psychoanalysis with the style of science.[26] Since Lacan, it can be said that the psychoanalytic clinic is not without the logical-mathematical formalization that characterizes scientific practice.

If only because of the most naïve and intuitive versions—and the least clinically operative—of the Oedipus complex, the castration complex, the unconscious, desire, the drives, and the *id*, the idea of an unknown knowledge has been incorporated in the West (perhaps one should only think of the "European" West) through the contributions of psychoanalysis. Psychoanalysis, however, is fundamentally different from other discourses that also maintain the impossibility of knowing everything, such as, among many others, those of religion, magic, and art, in that the latter do so through non-scientific means, such as mystical experience, revelation, suggestion, etc. In these practices, the unknown is always a name for the ineffable, which as such does not enable any analysis of the *particular way* in which lack-in-being constitutes the subject of science or habilitates the question of its relevance or the act that realizes it. The unknown is always a name for the ineffable, which, as such, prevents an analysis of the most particular inscription of the lack of being of the science's subject; further, it prevents us from raising the question of the relevance of such analysis and the act that would carry it out.

If science, as Lacan said, is an awakening, but a difficult and suspicious one, psychoanalysis is not a dream, but a reminder of the necessity of a *logico-formal* interpretation of dreams.[27]

Provided with this new logic, or a sketch of it, at least, Lacan radicalized psychoanalytic subversion. Among his followers, though, one observes a commitment similar to that of Freud: a forgetting of logic and, consequently, a return to a pure experience, the ineffable, and the poetic.

## Notes

1 Lacan, Jacques, *Seminar IV* (New York: Polity, 2022), p. 377.
2 Freud, Sigmund, "Project for a Scientific Psychology," (1950 [1985]) in *Standard Edition*, vol. 1.

3   Freud, Sigmund, "The Psychotherapy of Hysteria," in "Studies on Hysteria (1983–1895)," in *Standard Edition*, vol. 2.

4   Freud, Sigmund, "The Means of Representation in Dreams" in "The Interpretation of Dreams" (1900), in *Standard Edition*, vol. 4.

5   Freud, Sigmund, "On Dreams" (1901), in *Standard Edition*, vol. 5.

6   Freud, Sigmund, "The Antithetical Meaning of Primal Words" (1910), in *Standard Edition*, vol. 11.

7   Freud, Sigmund, "The Claims of Psychoanalysis to Scientific Interest" (1913), in *Standard Edition*, vol. 13.

8   Freud, Sigmund, "The Dream-Work" (1915), in *Standard Edition*, vol. 15.

9   Freud, Sigmund, "The Psychotherapy of Hysteria," in "Studies on Hysteria (1983–1895)," in *Standard Edition*, vol. 2, pp. 288–292; my underlining.

10  Derrida, Jacques, "The Structure, the Sign, and the Play in the Discourse of Human Sciences," in *Writing and Difference* (London and New York: Routledge and Kegan Paul, 1978).

11  Lacan, Jacques, "The Subversion of the Subject...," in *Écrits* (New York: Norton, 2006), pp. 673–796.

12  Cf. Lacan, Jacques, *Seminar XIV* (*The Logic of Phantasy* [*phantasme*]). *Staferla*. Especially the session of 12.21.1966.

13  Lacan, Jacques, *Seminar XI* (New York & London: Norton, 1981), p. 215.

14  Lacan, Jacques, *Seminar XI* (New York & London: Norton, 1981), p. 213.

15  Lacan, Jacques, "The Instance of the Letter...," in *Écrits* (New York: Norton, 2006).

16  Lacan, Jacques, "Position of the Unconscious...," in *Écrits* (New York: Norton, 2006), p. 714/842.

17  Lacan, Jacques, "Position of the Unconscious...," in *Écrits* (New York: Norton, 2006), p. 715/843.

18  Lacan, Jacques, *Seminar XI* (New York & London: Norton, 1981), p. 220.

19  Cf. Lacan, Jacques, *Seminar XIV* (*The Logic of Phantasy* [*phantasme*]). *Staferla*. Especially, sessions of 12.21.1966 and 01.11.1967.

20  Carlos Bermejo Mozas is incorrect when he claims that Lacan was the first to discover this logical operator (cf. http://www.carlosbermejo.net/logica%20pura/peirce1.htm). It was discovered by Henry Maurice Sheffer (1882–1964) in 1913. In fact, Charles Peirce had already discovered it in 1880, but his work was not published until 1933.

21  www.ucsm.edu.pe/rabarcat/, 1.2.2.6. Incompatibility.

22  Cf. Lacan, Jacques, *Seminar XIV*, session of 12.11.1966.

23  Cf. Chapter 7.c., "Cross-cap" in Eidelsztein, Alfredo, *Las estructuras clínicas a partir de Lacan*, vol. 1 (Buenos Aires: Letra Viva, 2008), pp. 228–232.

24  Cf. how Lacan closes his theoretical developments in *Seminar VII*.

25  Lacan, Jacques, "Of Structure as an Inmixing of an Otherness Prerequisite to Any Subject Whatever," in Macksey, Richard & Donato, Eugenio (eds.), *The Structuralist Controversy. The Languages of Criticism and the Sciences of Man* (Baltimore, MD and London: The Johns Hopkins University Press, 1979).

26  This is the exact opposite of the direction embraced by Jung, who made of the unconscious an eminently mystical, esoteric, and non-scientific instance.

27  Cf. Lacan, Jacques, *Séminaire XXIV*, session of 05.17.77.

# Part III

## Clinical Consequences

# Chapter 6

# *Ça parle* (It Speaks), *ça pense* (It Thinks), and Subjective Responsibility

It took 30 years for Lacan's followers to digest and assimilate their master's teaching. He is still misunderstood today, as he was in his time, which is why he always, especially toward the end of his life, declared that he had failed as a teacher of his own pupils, dissolving a few months before his death the school he had founded for that purpose.[1] However, those who purport to follow his work claim that his teaching has been elucidated. They do not understand his texts or his logic, so ultimately they read in Lacan exactly the same thing that Freud proposed. Accordingly, it seems appropriate that his self-proclaimed followers present themselves and are publicly known as "*Freudo*-Lacanians."

This process, which I designate as the "erasure of Lacan's subversion of the subject," has been carried out via different maneuvers. I distinguish at least four of them. The first consisted in supposing that Lacan's "return to Freud" meant a faithful return to the Freudian sources, which Lacan always rejected as a futile ideal.[2] Lacan's return implied, rather, turning Freud's theory on its head, i.e., inverting its orientation. In doing so, Lacan aimed to account for how a psychoanalysis based on his theory of the signifier could work.[3] The second was to assert that the new concepts proposed by Lacan were only modern names for old Freudian themes. This is what happened, for instance, with the notion of "subject," which came to be read as a new name for the individual. Likewise, for instance, the Other, i.e., A, was interpreted as the mother; the object a was equated with the object of the Freudian drive; and *jouissance* was read as Freudian pleasure and displeasure. The third was to reject and erase any notions that could not be reduced to Freud's theory, such as: structure, *mathème*, mathematical formalization, and topology. The fourth consisted of a more subtle maneuver: they claimed that a very important set of Lacan's conceptual inventions can be found in Freud's work. Such is the case of the subject-matter of this essay: *ça pense* (it thinks) and *ça parle* (it speaks), which Freud never maintained. However, the Freudo-Lacanians effortlessly claim that these ideas were actually defended by Freud. Thus, they feel no need to ask why Lacan may have introduced to psychoanalysis such surprising assertions that are absolutely alien to the spirit of Freudian theory and to the prevailing ideology within and beyond the psychoanalytic domain.

DOI: 10.4324/9781003485339-9

What is literally *unbelievable* of Lacan's proposal can be expressed as follows: the "subject" of thinking and speaking is not *someone* but an *it*. Or, in a self-contradictory manner, the "who" is an "it." For Lacan, *ça parle* and *ça pense* are absolutely necessary in order to understand how psychoanalytic practice functions, operates, and heals in its specific modality and ethics.

In a very general manner, the system of differences between Freud's and Lacan's theories can be summed up this way: according to Freud, the *id*, *das Es*, though it indicates something impersonal, a "non-ego," comes from within the three-dimensional biological body and occupies the place of the kernel of our being, *das Kern unseres Wesen*, which, similar to Schopenhauer's earlier proposition,[4] Freud defined, at the end of his life, as follows:

> The core of our being, then, is formed by the obscure *id* [...] Within this *id* the organic drives operate, [...] compounded of fusions of two primal forces (*Eros* and destructiveness) in varying proportions and are differentiated from one another by their relation to organs and systems of organs.[5]

Freud's conception is a moment of a historical, theoretical, and philosophical dispute in the West. This debate, which has been going on for at least eight centuries and is still largely unknown, pertains to whether or not a primal three-dimensional substance, a body of flesh and blood, is required to yield and create thought and speech.

As will be shown later in this essay, Lacan defends a view that has historical precedents to some extent in, among others, Saint Augustine, Averroes, G.C. Lichtenberg, F.W.J. Schelling, F. Nietzsche, C. Lévi-Strauss, P. Ricoeur, and M. Angenot. Lacan claims, "[...] *ça pense en moi* (*Es denkt in mir*)": It thinks in me.[6] The opposite—the prevailing view in the West—is that each of us, individually, do the thinking.

Thus, for Lacan, contrary to Freud, it (*ça*) thinks alone, steadily, autonomously, and independently of all biological life. A three-dimensional substance working as the source, the original spring for thinking, is not required. As Freud states in "Moral Responsibility for the Content of Dreams," much cited by the Freudo-Lacanians (one of the circles in the West that most decisively upholds the notion of "individual responsibility"), one is not even within the psychoanalytic domain if one fails to take individual moral responsibility for one's unconscious thoughts.[7] This is undoubtedly why, when they engage in the juridical debate about legal responsibility and accountability, Freudo-Lacanians tend to favor the imprisonment of criminals.

For Lacan, "'it' thinks alone...and it thinks steadily."[8] The specificity of his conception of the psychoanalytic subject lies in this claim. For Freud, there cannot be thought without someone doing the thinking. Thus, a fundamental element of Lacan's teaching has not yet been admitted: "We don't speak to the subject. 'It' speaks of it."[9]

On the contrary, Freud maintained that one is responsible for what one thinks and does. Indeed, he argues, there is first an individual animal body endowed with specific drives, the adhesiveness of personal libido, and experiences of direct satisfaction and dissatisfaction, each inscribed within itself by means of singular representations that, at a later time, once they cross the barrier of repression, become associated with words that traverse the superego and enable its thoughts.[10]

According to Lacan, following his theory of the signifier, the postulation "It thinks alone" prevents even the logical possibility of plagiarism, since for him no one can own thought.[11] Further, he simply proposes that there is no intellectual property, which he considers to be a real prejudice.[12] Thoughts are thought by "it" (*ça*). This is how he criticizes and re-elaborates Freud's drive-like *id* [*ello pulsional*].

Freud's stance, like that of most psychoanalysts, is designated by Alain de Libera as "attributism," which, as he argues in his work on the archaeology of the subject (mandatory reading for any psychoanalyst), necessarily ends in the positing of a responsible subject, and, in later modernity, of a subject susceptible to being legally accused.[13] From this it follows that if there is no one who can be legally accused, there is no subject. In this reasoning, we notice the insistent echoes of the Freudo-Lacanians on "subjective responsibility," an expression that never appears in Lacan's corpus. Let us also notice that the reasons they qualify responsibility as "subjective" are not at all clear. Do they, perhaps, want to suggest that there is a non-individual notion of responsibility?

As affirmed throughout his work (for instance, in "The Function and Field of Speech and Language in Psychoanalysis," "Variations on the Standard Treatment," "On a Question Prior to Any Possible Treatment of Psychosis" and "The Third"), for Lacan, responsibility in psychoanalysis is applicable only to the psychoanalyst. This is the exact meaning of his claim, "one is always responsible for one's position as a subject."[14] Interestingly enough, this is the quotation most cited by Freudo-Lacanians when they argue for the *opposite* claim.

My position rests on four observations:

1  The paragraph containing the quotation deploys Lacan's thesis that psychoanalysis operates with the "subject *of science*."
2  He does *not* claim that we are always responsible for our position as subjects (in the plural).
3  The French term translated as "position" is *position*, which originates in *poser*: to formulate, posit, or propose. Lacan claims that the formulation and positing of the psychoanalytic subject is the analyst's. And
4  Regarding the analysand, Lacan's position is very clear: the notion of unconscious contradicts that of subjective responsibility.

To understand Lacan's insights, it is necessary to return to a fundamental difference derived from his conception of the signifier. For Lacan, the sign always implies someone, since "...the sign represents something to someone...."[15] However, the signifier, in its specificity, since it belongs to no one, establishes that there is no one responsible for anything.[16] In his seminar at the beginning of the last decade of his theoretical production he puts it in remarkably categorical and challenging terms:

> This is actually what Freud discovered in fact around 1920 [i.e., around the time when "Beyond the Pleasure Principle" was published; AE], and here, in a way, is the point at which his discovery backtracks.
>
> His discovery was to have spelled out the unconscious, and I defy any-one to say that this can be anything other than the remark that there is a perfectly articulated knowledge for which strictly speaking no subject is responsible. When a subject happens to encounter it all of a sudden, to come upon this knowledge he was not expecting, good God, he—he who speaks—finds himself very confused indeed.[17]

Thus, most psychoanalysts clearly read Lacan's teaching backward. Their stance is also contrary to the following argument, one that is never raised (not only by psychoanalysts, but also by the general public, as our society, individualistic as it is, has created the figure of the modern genius who develops his discoveries in absolute isolation: Marx, Freud, Einstein, etc., count, in this view, as eminent examples of geniuses): if it is not the case that it is "that" (*ça*) which thinks, and thinks in a way that remains separate from each particular individual, how is it that in the history of science there are so many cases in which several researchers arrive at the same discovery at the same time, with no knowledge of each other? To cite just a few cases that should become widely known: the theory of relativity, which was proposed simultaneously and baptized with the same name by Albert Einstein and Henri Poincaré, (although with disparate arguments); the theory of evolution, by Charles Darwin and Alfred Wallace; infinitesimal calculus by Gottfried Leibniz and Isaac Newton; the breathing mechanism explained in the same year by Priestly, Scheele, Lavoisier, Spallanzani and Davy; the Möbius band discovered simultaneously by August Möbius and Johann Listing and, lastly, the solution to the problem of the formal justification of Euclid's fifth postulate, discovered in the same years, and more than two millennia after it was posed, by Nicolai Lobachevsky, Janos Bolyay, and Carl Gauss. There is a myriad of other cases already compiled and widely available, even on the internet. To my mind, all this indicates that *ça pense* only in a given society at a particular historical time. Thus, it becomes possible for a plurality of individuals to express it.

Lacan's conceptualizations of *ça pense* and *ça parle* coincide in his teaching in that both entail the radical rejection of "I speak" and "I think" as the Cartesian origin and foundation of Western modernity. For Lacan, psychoanalysis proposes to its society and epoch, and this on the basis of its particular way of "handling" the unconscious, that the personal ego, as an individual and internal source and origin of thinking and speaking should be rejected.

However, *ça pense* and *ça parle* are not identical. Lacan says, "*Ça parle* in [the] place of the Other [A]," which must be understood as a key element in Lacan's attempt to rectify Freud's theory by means of developing a new theory of the subject.[18] This could be said more precisely as follows: "If the Other [A] is the locus of speech, it is there where it speaks [...]."[19] Let us recall that Lacan, going against the most common conception of human communication, always posited that one does not emit but receives one's own message in an inverted form from the Other (A).

Thus, to account for the structure of this conceptual field in Lacan's teaching, one must distinguish among three interrelated concepts: unconscious, Other [A], and it [*ça*]. Their articulation is as follows: the unconscious is posited as the locus of speech and conceived as Other, A, for each particular subject. Further, the unconscious *is* where *it* speaks. Since it is also the case that "...truth founds itself in it...,"[20] one may conclude that "I [*moi*], truth, speak,"[21] alone and autonomously.

It follows that in analytic practice no one *confesses* the truth, as the latter speaks from and by itself on its own account. Psychoanalysis, so understood, i.e., as long as the analyst operates with the signifying subject and does not admit the idea of subjective responsibility, is not a "soul police," a device whose nature and aims coincide with that of Christian religion.

These theses, which in psychoanalysis have only been defended by Lacan, require that one posits the *parlêtre* (not, as his followers translate, the "speaking-being") as the necessary creator of truth. The *parlêtre* is both a creation of language and a being-spoken-by-language, and this is why it is always being-spoken from a locus different from the one it thinks it is spoken.[22] Lacan formulates his own position as an analyst as follows: "I do not ask myself, 'who speaks?'; I ask myself, 'from where does it speak?'"[23]

As for the *ça pense*, it should be stressed that Lacan's proposal is entirely contrary to Freud's: "...there is only one *cogitatum* [that which is thought], and it entails no ego...."[24] According to this logic, as stated above, plagiarism is impossible, since there is no such thing as intellectual property.[25] At least within analytic practice, Lacan never admits that there is an ego doing the thinking.

In Lacan's psychoanalytic logic, then, Descartes' *cogito* must be entirely rewritten. Only Lacan, holding in place the function of the *it* [*ça*], rejects both the "I think" and the "I am" as its alleged logical consequence. He writes, "...it thinks there, where it is impossible that the subject articulates the 'therefore I am'."[26]

For Lacan, only *ça* thinks, and this defines his ethical stance. It is by articulating this thesis with his positing of the unconscious as unknown knowledge that he can write, "...*ça pense* without ever being able to know it...," without ever recovering itself as a self-consciousness ("I think")—It thinks without knowing it."[27] It cannot know it, but, as "...it is not ineffable, because *ça* speaks...," it *can* be known and analyzed.[28]

Thus, as already shown in the previous discussion of the claim that the unconscious is the locus of the Other, A, Lacan resumes the debate between those who argue that "someone thinks" (the position of Freud, among many others) and those who defend the idea that "*ça pense* in me" (for instance, Nietzsche and Lévi-Strauss). Lacan, arguing for the latter, adds something crucial to the debate, namely, the notion that *ça pense* in the locus of the Other, A, for the subject. In my view, it is only by embracing this thesis—still unknown and therefore unrecognized—that psychoanalysis can find its specificity as a theory and as a practice.

Finally, Freudo-Lacanians, clinging to the notion of subjective responsibility, once again interpreted "Wo Es was, soll Ich werden" as Freud and the post-Freudians did. In Freud's words:

> Nevertheless, it may be admitted that the therapeutic efforts of psycho-analysis have chosen a similar line of approach. Its intention is, indeed, to strengthen the ego, make it more independent of the super-ego, to widen its field of perception and enlarge its organization, so that it can appropriate fresh portions of the *id*. Where *id* was, there ego shall be.[29]

Lacan substituted the latter for "Where it was, the subject shall be."[30] Here we see a substitution of Freud's ego for the signifying subject and of the German *Imperfekt* for the French Imperfect tense: what shall be will come from a place where it was not yet.[31] More clearly: the subject, who is no-one, shall come from where *ça pense* and *ça parle*, which is a place where things are not yet.

## Notes

1   Eidelsztein, Alfredo, "El fracaso de Lacan" en *El rey está desnudo* 2 and 3 (Buenos Aires: Letra Viva, 2009 and 2010).
2   Lacan, Jacques, *Seminar XIII*, session of 06.01.1966. Staferla, p. 641.
3   Lacan, Jacques, "Ouverture de la section clinique," in *Ornicar?*, 9, avril 1977, pp. 7–14.
4   Schopenhauer, Arthur, *The World as World and Representation* (New York: Dover, 1969).
5   Freud, Sigmund, "An Outline of Psycho-Analysis," in *Standard Edition 23*, p. 199.
6   de Libera, Alain, *Archéologie du sujet, vol.1. Naissance du sujet* (Paris: Librairie Phylosophique J. Vrin, 2007), p. 35.
7   Cf. Freud, Sigmund, "Some Additional Notes on Dream-Interpretation as a Whole," section B, in *Standard Edition 19*, pp. 127–138.
8   Lacan, Jacques, "On a Question Prior to Any Possible Treatment of Psychosis," in *Écrits* (New York: Norton, 2006), p. 458/548.
9   Lacan, Jacques, "Position of the Unconscious," in *Écrits* (New York: Norton, 2006), p. 708/835.
10  Freud, Sigmund, "Analysis Terminable and Interminable," in Standard Edition *23*, p. 241.
11  Lacan, Jacques, *Seminar XIII*. Session of 03.23.1966. *Staferla*, p. 377.
12  Lacan, Jacques, "Response to Jean Hyppolite's Commentary on Freud's 'Verneinung'," in *Écrits* (New York: Norton, 2006), p. 329/395. He also defends this position in *Seminar XIII*. Session of 03.23.1966. *Staferla*, p. 375.
13  de Libera, Alain, *Archéologie du sujet, vol.1. Naissance du sujet* (Paris: Librairie Phylosophique J. Vrin, 2007), pp. 100ff.
14  Lacan, Jacques, "Science and Truth," in *Écrits* (New York: Norton, 2006), p. 729/859.
15  Lacan, Jacques, *Seminar IX*. Session of 01.24.1962. *Staferla*, p. 171.

16  Lacan, Jacques, "Geneva Lecture on the Symptom," in *Analysis 1*, January 1989, pp. 7–26, p. 15.

17  Lacan, Jacques, *S17*, p. 77/89.

18  Lacan, Jacques, "Les noms du pére." *Seminar X*. Session of 11.20.1963, unpublished.

19  Lacan, Jacques, *Seminar V*. Session of 06.25.1958, p. 334.

20  Lacan, Jacques, "Science and Truth," in *Écrits* (New York: Norton, 2006), pp. 579/690.

21  Lacan, Jacques, *Seminar XVI*. Session of 11.13.1968. *Staferla*, p. 16.

22  Lacan, Jacques, *Seminar XII*. Session of 02.18.1975. *Staferla*, p. 118.

23  Lacan, Jacques, *Seminar XXIII*. Session of 01.26.1966. *Staferla*, p. 253.

24  Cf. Lacan, Jacques, *Seminar XIX*. Session of 11.19.1958. *Staferla*, p. 54.

25  Lacan, Jacques, "Response to Jean Hyppolite's Commentary on Freud's 'Vermeinung,'" in *Écrits* (New York: Norton, 2006), pp. 318–333, pp. 328–329. Cf., also, Lacan's *Seminar XIII*, session of 03.23.1966. *Staferla*, p. 375, and *Seminar XVI*, session of 11.20.68. *Staferla*, p. 16.

26  Lacan, Jacques, "C'est à la lecture de Freud," in *Pas-tout Lacan*, p. 1873. Online resource: https://ecole-lacanienne.net/wp-content/uploads/2016/04/1926-1981-Pas-tout-Lacan.pdf (last accessed: September 15, 2024).

27  Lacan, Jacques, "C'est à la lecture de Freud," in *Pas-tout Lacan*, p. 1873.

28  Lacan, Jacques, "On a Question Prior to All Possible Treatment of Psychosis," in *Écrits* (New York: Norton, 2006), p. 480/577.

29  Freud, Sigmund, "New Introductory Lectures to Psychoanalysis," *Conference 31*, *Standard Edition 22*, p. 80.

30  Cf., for instance, "The Subversion of the Subject and the Dialectic of Desire in the Freudian Unconscious" and "The Instance of the Letter in the Unconscious, or Reason Since Freud," in *Écrits* (New York: Norton, 2006), pp. 671/793–702/828 and pp. 412/493–444/530.

31  Cf., for instance, *Seminar XV*. Session of 01.10.1968. *Staferla*, pp. 97–98.

# Chapter 7

# Sex, Gender, and Sexuality in Lacanian Perspective[1]

Freud's views, at least the fundamental ones, penetrated deeply into modern Western sensibility. Or, conversely, Freudian views were reliable, amplified expressions of certain conceptions of his society and time, i.e., Europe at the end of the nineteenth century. It was a period of significant transformations in ways of thinking about the real, truth, authority, family, art, etc. Such transformations were fundamentally driven by the formal sciences, undergoing a veritable Big Bang in those same spatial and temporal coordinates, but also by the simultaneous advance of democracy and individual rights, the unbridled progress of capitalism, the development of technologies that unexpectedly altered daily life, and the secularization of key areas of social life. All of this led to a real and inevitable clash and to an ideological conflict that left no one indifferent and unaffected.

With regard to such a conflict—which played out on a global scale and which, broadly speaking, could perhaps be equated with modernity—I propose that the multiple responses to it can be read in two ways, depending on whether they are aligned with one of the following opposing tendencies. On the one hand, there is a tendency toward higher scientific abstraction, further dissolution of supposed material reality, increased undermining of traditional authority, and greater distrust in personal experience and all that is provided by the senses. This position wants to venture into the new, even if, or specially because, it is yet unknown to us. On the other hand, the quite opposite attitude consists in returning to past ways of living, strengthening traditional authority, prioritizing individual lived-experiences, distrusting pure intellect and mathematical abstractions, advocating a return to the customary form of the nuclear family, etc. These alternatives can therefore be posited as either moving toward the ignored future or returning to the well-known past.

Freud's psychoanalysis conceived of itself as revolutionary and presented itself to society as such, much like Nazism and Communism, which, I propose, can also be considered attempts to solve the unavoidable political conflict that arose in nineteenth century Europe. Indeed, in its beginnings it was customary to consider Freudian psychoanalysis revolutionary. Over time, however, many scholars began to identify and to denounce its conservative aspects. This denunciation would later become standard practice. My position is that Freudian theory is an enormous theoretical corpus that, despite its scientific and subversive presentation, consistently

DOI: 10.4324/9781003485339-10

assumes a position oriented toward a return to the past. This is a consequence of its explicit axiological commitments: the old notions of authority, father, woman, science, and the like are considered better than the new ones. On the other hand, Lacan, remaining within psychoanalysis, assumes the opposite position: his work abandons all the beliefs that, though they prevailed in their socio-cultural time, have been shown to be false by modern science: the male is more valuable than the female, the universe has a center, personal experience is not deceptive, drives are biological, everything is demonstrable, etc. If one remains within the Freudian position, it is simply impossible to conceive of and operate with the specific problems, pleasures, and suffering of what Lacan rightly calls "the subject of science."

According to Freud, the normality of the maturation process of each individual consists in the confluence of gender identity and biology—as is well known, he maintained that "anatomy is destiny."[2] Thus, it is both normal and expected that the male becomes a boy and the female a girl. Although he recognizes that this is not always the case, this would be, in Freud's theory, the ideal evolutionary process for every individual of the human species in any society and culture. Since for Freud sexual maturation culminates in "the choice of a sexual object," he must account for the process by which each human being arrives at or should arrive at this choice, a process wherein sexual identity is determined by the biological domain. The "machine" that yields such a result is, in his view, the Oedipus Complex, which, once traversed, makes of us boys or girls depending on our biological constitutions (being male or female). Later in his research, Freud would admit a quota of homosexuality even in "normal" cases. Either way, for the Oedipus Complex to yield the expected result, the female mother and the male father must fulfil sex-specific roles within the family in the child's early life. Since this is considered a normal result, Freud must also specify the universal properties of masculinity and the femininity. Thus, the man must be dominant, since the male libido is active, and the woman must be dominated, since hers is passive. It follows that a man's fulfillment results from his active and judicious management, transformation, and mastery of reality. Quite differently, the fulfillment of women, whom Freud conceives of as more passionate than men, takes place inside the home, having and raising children. The strong superego of the former enables him to perform a social function, whereas the weak superego of the latter prevents or should prevent her from doing so.

The phallus, a fundamental element of the Freudian Oedipus, is the symbol of power and action, and is therefore admired and coveted. Thus, men fear losing it—castration anxiety—and women feel the detriment of not having it—their penis envy. Accordingly, if a woman is too active and powerful, or seeks to be so, she should be reprimanded for being or behaving like a "phallic woman." In all fairness, let us notice that the latter was not affirmed by Freud himself, but by some of his disciples, who developed his ideas.

Because these conceptions are still with us, being lesbian, gay, bisexual, transgender, queer, intersex, asexual, etc., generates guilt, not only in "perverts," but also in their parents, including those with no psychoanalytic background whatsoever.

Again, such positions are the result of a *failure* and *deviation* in the Oedipal process and, consequently, of the roles of the father and the mother.

From a completely different perspective Lacan holds that "man," "woman," and "child" are only signifiers:

> There isn't the slightest prediscursive reality, for the very fine reason that what constitutes a collectivity—what I called men, women, and children—means nothing qua prediscursive reality. Men, women, and children are but signifiers.[3]

In his theoretical model this implies at least two fundamental considerations: (a) as such, these signifiers mean nothing in themselves, since they consist only in the difference they hold from all others, and (b) if they are signifiers, they have no relation to either nature or biology. Lacan's formula, "There is no sexual relation" (*Il n'y a pas de rapport sexuel*) affirms precisely the impossibility of matching "man" with male, "woman" with female, and "child" with human offspring. Naturally, there are sexual practices, but the alleged natural sexual condition of the signifier's subject has been lost from the beginning and forever.

Accordingly, the paternal metaphor is, for Lacan, the "machine" that accounts for how the only fundamental law is inscribed in each story: no representative of A (the place of language, logic, and truth), that is, no Other could ever coincide with it. The function of the paternal metaphor is to legislate for each case that *Other ≠ A*. Neither mothers, fathers, grandparents, nor any natural instance of a representation of authority that has operated in a particular story can arrogate to themselves the power of language, which, although it is inherently "not everything" (A̸), is the only source of power [*potencia*]. Thus, if the "machine" operated in its specific function, there would be no omnipotent instance. The paternal metaphor will also end up giving *meaning* to the subject (never a definitive one), but not a sexual identity as in Freud's theory of Oedipus. The "Mother's Desire" does not refer to the mother, but to the incarnation of the Other (who could be a mother, a father, a couple of mothers or fathers, etc.). Retroactively, we can determine that the "Name-of-the-Father" has operated in its specific function if the source of power (always, ultimately, the power of language) has not coincided with the father or with anyone else. The law instituted by the "Name-of-the-Father" is the one that affirms that no one can embody or hold the law by himself.

Lacan derives these designations, "Mother" and "Father," from Indo-European history.[4] In this language, a clear distinction is made between "Pater," a pure mythological function (as in the case of *Ius Pater*: Jupiter, exclusively a name), and "father," the relative who nourishes. "Mother" is also distinguished from the nourishing relative, as shown in the expression "Mother Earth." In this system, the fraternal bond (*Frater*) is different from the relationship between two people resulting from their having been engendered in the same womb (*Adelphos*). Thus, *Pater, Mater*, and *Frater* do not designate father, mother, and brother. Furthermore, all epochs and societies suffer from a specific kind of deception emerging from the false incarnations of the function "Name-of-the-Father:" King, High Priest,

Master, Father with parental authority, revolutionary leader, and even (at least in the West, given the ubiquitous presence of the life sciences) the selfish gene, etc. According to Lacan, as contexts and signifying articulations change, so too does the Name-of-the-Father, which is why it must be replaced by the Names-of-the-Father, a *plural* that, in turn, forces us to conceive different symbolic orders. For Lacan, it is not a question of moving from geocentrism to heliocentrism, from the mother of Oedipus to the father—it is rather a question of embracing the non-existence of *any* center in *any* symbolic order. A partial historical instantiation of this is Kepler's (not Copernicus') revolution, through which the elliptical orbits of the planets were established. According to Kepler, in one focus of the ellipse there is the Sun and, in the other, there is nothing.

In Lacan's work, "phallus" takes on many meanings. In the context of our discussion, let us remark that the phallus inscribes the fundamental property of the signifier: there is nothing natural in the sexual. In other words, it is impossible to eliminate the presence of the *Aidos*, the devil of modesty or the deity of dignity. These mark the sexual domain, human sexuality, precisely in virtue of their non-natural, signifying origin. We see their ordinary manifestations in, for example, modesty or disgust, which signal a "limit" that does not exist in the natural domain. That sexuality is entirely an effect of the signifier is verified too in the fact that sexuality is unthinkable without the existence of phenomena such as rituals, wearing veils, clothing, adornments, privacy, darkness, money, etc.

In every story, whether of a subject, a family, or a people, signifiers function not only as pure differences, but are also woven into *chains*. So localized in a particular signifying chain, they lose their condition of absolute fluidity. Some of them repeat and insist, so they are susceptible to being identified and communicated. When the latter takes place, it is because the signifiers that comprise the chains have been transformed into, and determined as, *letters*. For Lacan, a letter is the state that a signifier acquires when it is localized in a signifying chain. For this reason, it receives a lasting meaning, which, although it will always refer to other signifiers and not to an empirical object, is stable for a period of time—at least as long as the relevant linguistic, family, and socio-cultural *context* does not fundamentally change.

From this perspective it is possible to investigate and establish what values and meanings "woman," "man," and "child" acquire in a given context. These are obviously in constant transformation—they will change faster is some contexts than in others—which means that when the analyst diagnoses them, he must focus more on determining those changes than on contrasting them with allegedly constant identities. Some of these changes require rectification, solution, or cure because of the excessive suffering they bring. In our time and society, such suffering can lead to a demand for psychoanalytic treatment.

Contrary to Freud, Lacan does not work with the notion of male or female libido. Furthermore, there is nothing in Lacan's theory like a libido understood as energy originating from inside the anatomical body. Moreover, the drive, i.e., "the echo in the body of the fact that there is a saying," is posited and written as T.

This is a formula that contains no biological element, as all its elements, including the bodily "hole," originate in the signifier. *Jouissance*, in turn, is the *jouissance* of the Other, jA, which indicates that it is not anybody's *jouissance*. Finally, phallic *jouissance*, j□, must be read as "localized" "outside the body," which is in total discontinuity with any biological, patriarchal, or sexist conceptions of sex, sexuality, and the body. Similarly, Freud's psychic apparatus is singular and internal to an individual, properties that are not applicable to Lacan's articulation of the symbolic, the imaginary, and the real, which constitute a structure.

From this perspective, Lacan's formulas of sexuation may be interpreted as his diagnosis, in our time and culture, of how "man" and "woman," as signifiers, have become letters, which he presents in terms of the following terms and functions: male, female, S(A̶), $, objet *a*, Φ, *L̶a* , and their reciprocal articulations.

Given that Lacan writes these functions in an algebraic manner, it is plausible that he considers that it is possible to interpret how the signifiers "man" and "woman" have been translated into letters in every era and every society. In each particular context, what "man" and "woman" mean, as letters, will be different.

Lacan's concept of "subject," defined as, "what a signifier represents in relation to another signifier," necessarily implies that it is not a man, a woman, or a child; further, it is not gay, lesbian, trans, bisexual, neurotic, etc.: it simply *is not*. It lacks being and identity. In each particular history of a person, a family, or a people, the value of "subject" participates in signifying networks, chains of chains, in which it acquires multiple meanings whose truth and permanence are never fixed. Which of those meanings we confront and reject with utter indignation and which we help to thrive depends on our ethics, though we should never lose sight of the fact that the issue is ultimately in nobody's hands. The same is applicable to the signifiers "Islamic," "Gypsy," "Black," "Jew," "Yankee," "refugee," "Israeli," etc. These signifiers do not emerge from any objective stance, neither that of the biological body, nor that of any reliable, measurable statistics, and thus they have no identity or ontological consistency. The meaning they receive derives from the historical articulation of the signifying framework in each case and from the position they assume in it.

"Psychoanalyst" does not designate anything in itself either its meaning depends on each case and each context. Not every psychoanalyst is patriarchal, sexist, and Eurocentric. Just as there is no one linguistics, one philosophy, or one physics (there are multiple linguistic, philosophical, and physical theories within each of these fields), there is no one discourse of psychoanalysis: there are many, some of them still unknown in mainstream circles, as is perhaps the one elaborated in these lines. Either way, they should not be ignored. To affirm that psychoanalysis is a unified field is to uphold the same epistemological defect as that of binarism, racism, or xenophobia. It is the responsibility of each analyst and each society of analysts to determine what kind of psychoanalysis is assumed, practiced, and disseminated, and in this, to begin with, whether it is "Freudian" or not, paternalistic or not, biological and individualistic or not, etc.

It is possible that Lacan's work has not succeeded in totally rejecting the Eurocentric, sexist, and patriarchal legacy that can be located in Freud's work.

A position that prioritizes difference must make of this its eminent task. If we do so, our very first axiom should be: first, there is language, history, the Other, society, and culture, and then, *only then*, there are the multiple ways in which bodies can be or have been inscribed, ways in which suffering and *jouissance* affect us, and, correlatively, point toward the positions and healing resources that we must either assume or reject.

*

As an annex, I would like to add a few brief observations to Paul B. Preciado, Jean-Claude Maleval, and Jacques-Alain Miller.

1  *To Paul B. Preciado.* Psychoanalysis cannot be identified with Freudism. Not all psychoanalytic theories are Freudian. There is at least a version of Lacan's theory that is not conceive of sex and sexual difference as ultimately founded in anatomical differences. This version of Lacan's theory posits a Big Bang of language and discourse, which entails the rejection of all non-discursive, i.e., natural and bodily causation.

2  *To Jean-Claude Maleval.* Regardless of any alleged "law" formulated by Lacan or any other psychoanalyst, the fact remains that we don't know whether there will be an infinite amount of *jouissance*, though we do know that there will be infinite modalities of *jouissance*—a *jouissance* that is not pre-discursive. "There is *jouissance*" and "its modalities are not infinite" are, taken as mere assertions, prejudices. If there are to be asserted as what they really are, namely, theses, they should be proven.

3  *To Jacques-Alain Miller.* The vindication of so-called "trans rights" is not the latest trend in the United States: it is an expression of liberal democracy and human rights. Non-trans people also suffer from being certain (even without knowing it) of their sexual identity (A = A). They don't necessarily question their identity more than trans folks. As for the number of psychotic cases in the trans community: how to determine what that number is? That non-trans people believe that they are more sane than trans folks is not a criterion we can simply accept as valid for psychoanalytic theory and practice. Such beliefs are only prejudices.

## Notes

1  Original title: "Diversas posiciones psicoanalíticas respecto del sexo, el género, y la sexualidad. Contribución a un posible debate con Paul B. Preciado, Jean-Claude Maleval, y Jacques-Alain, Miller." The article was a response to Preciado's intervention at the meeting of the *École de la Cause Freudienne* of November 17, 2019: "Mujeres en Psicoanálisis" [*Women in Psychoanalysis*]. An extended version was included in Preciado's book, *Yo soy el monstruo que os habla: informe para una academia de psicoanalistas* (Barcelona: Anagrama, 2020). My essay aims to contribute to the debate between Preciado and Maleval, Jean-Claude, who responded to Preciado in his "Cuando Preciado interpela al psicoanálisis" (December, 1, 2019, available here: https://lacanquotidien.fr/

blog/wp-content/uploads/2019/12/LQ-856.pdf). Miller, Jacques-Alain (with Catherine Millot) joined the debate with the essay, "La question trans dans la psychanalyse et pour le psychanalyste," in *Figures de la psychanalyse*, 2022/2021, 43, pp. 151–161.

2 Freud, Sigmund, "The Dissolution of the Oedipus Complex," in *Standard Edition 19*, p. 178.

3 Lacan, Jacques. *Seminar XX*. Session of 01.09.1973.

4 Cf. Benveniste, Émile, *Vocabulaire des institutions indoeuropéennes, tome I* (Paris: Éditions de Minuit, 1969).

# Part IV

# Appendix

Appendix

# Chapter 8

# Brief Presentation of the Big Bang Theory

One can think of the big bang, as conceptualized by the theoretical model or models that sustain it, as the moment in which all matter emerged from nothingness or emptiness, i.e., as an account of the possible origin of the universe. At that moment, matter, a point of infinite density that lacked volume, "exploded," generating thereby its expansion in all directions and creating what we know today as the universe. In this view the universe is dynamically conceived of as having a history and no longer as an eternal being. Not only matter and energy, but also time and space, or space-time, began with the big bang.

To understand better the conditions for this absolute beginning, one can think as follows: the universe originated from one point of zero dimensions and infinite energy, a point with no volume and infinitely high temperature, which we should not think of as being at the center of anything or as a grain of sand.

In cosmological physics, the theory of the big explosion is a scientific model aiming to explain the origin of the universe and its subsequent development, starting from a spatio-temporal singularity. This model is based on a collection of solutions for the equations of Einstein's general relativity theory. Although these equations do not constitute a complete theory, the model has ample observational support and highly predictive power.

The term "big bang" is used to refer both to the moment in which the observable expansion of the universe began (everything that existed and took place prior to it remains unobservable) and, more generally, to the cosmological paradigm that explains the origin and expansion of the universe. The term "big bang" may be misleading. Indeed, at the beginning of the universe there was no explosion and it was not, consequently, big: the universe emerged out of an infinitely small "singularity," followed by the beginning and expansion of space, time, and the emergence of matter.

At the core of the big bang, there is the idea that the theory of general relativity can be combined with the observations of large-scale isotropy (i.e., the quality of bodies whose physical properties do not depend on direction) and homogeneity in the distribution of galaxies and the changes in their relative position, which allows to determine the conditions of the universe along the timeline.

DOI: 10.4324/9781003485339-12

The big bang theory is the result of the work of many scientists from different disciplines, all of them with a robust mathematical background. The genesis of this theoretical model goes back to the works of A. Friedman and G. Lemaître who, in 1922 and 1927 respectively, used the theory of relativity to demonstrate that the universe is continually moving and expanding. A few years later, in 1929, astronomer E. Hubble found that galaxies located beyond the Milky Way moved away as if the universe was in constant expansion. In 1948, physicist G. Gamow posited that the universe was created out of a big explosion (the big bang). Recently, spatial satellites launched into orbit were able to detect the traces of this "gigantic, primal explosion," but one should stress that we won't ever be able to "see" or "hear" what preceded it.

The big bang theory was developed from theoretical developments and extraordinary observations. It is because of the latter that, since the beginning of the twentieth century, we know that most spiral nebulae are moving away from the earth. Originally, though, the cosmological implications of these observations were not drawn; neither were they inferred from the fact that the alleged nebulae were in fact galaxies external to the Milky Way.

Besides, A. Einstein's theory of general relativity (developed in the second decade of the twentieth century) does not admit of static solutions (i.e., the universe must be either expanding or contracting), a result that Einstein himself considered to be wrong and attempted to mend by introducing the cosmological constant. The first scientist to formally apply relativity theory to cosmology putting aside the cosmological constant was A. Friedman, whose equations posit that the universe can expand or contract.

Working independently between 1927 and 1930, G. Lamaître obtained the same equations and proposed, on the basis of the spiral nebulae's recession, that the universe started with the explosion of a primal atom—a point.

In 1929, E. Hubble made observations that allowed him to corroborate Lemaître's theory. He proved that the spiral nebulae are in fact galaxies and measured its distances, observing variable stars in distant galaxies. He discovered that galaxies move away from each other at a speed directly proportional to their distance.

According to the cosmological principle, the moving away of galaxies suggested that the universe was expanding. From this idea, two opposing hypotheses arose. The first was Lemaître's big bang theory, supported and developed by G. Gamow. The second was F. Hoyle's model for the stationary state theory, according to which new matter is generated as galaxies move away from each other. In the latter model, the universe is fundamentally the same at every given moment in time. For many years, each theory captivated a similar number of supporters.

Over time, though, observational evidence supported the idea that the universe evolved from an infinitely dense, hot, and volume-less state. Since the discovery of microwave background radiation in 1965, the big bang is regarded as the best theory to explain the origin and evolution of the cosmos. In the 1960s, S. Hawking and others proved that the singularity is an essential component of gravity in

Einstein's theory. As a result, the vast majority of cosmologists accepted the big bang theory and the universe was conceived as being finite in time.

As a result of significant progress in telescopic technology and all the data gathered by the COBE satellite and the Hubble and WMAP spatial telescopes, by the end of the 1990s major progress in the big bang cosmology took place. This data allowed cosmologists to calculate many of the big bang parameters with a high degree of precision and conclude that the expansion of the universe seems to be accelerating.

Based on measurements of the universe's expansion as they result from the observations of 1a-type supernovas (the focus of which are [a] the variation of the temperature in different scales in microwave background radiation and [b] the correlation among galaxies), the age of the universe is estimated to be a bit over 13.5 billion years. It is remarkable that many measurements proceeding independently from each other, coincide, which constitutes strong evidence for the so-called "Concordance Cosmological Model."

Einstein's gravitational theory predicts that "at the first instant" there must be a gravitational singularity of infinite density. Aiming to solve this physical paradox, scientists propose that it is necessary to develop a theory of quantum gravity. The understanding of this phase of the universe's history is one of the major unsolved problems in physics, one that is currently being actively tackled by contemporary cosmologists.

The big bang is not an explosion of matter that expands to fill out an empty universe. It is the very space-time continuum—that which expands itself. And it is its expansion that causes an increase in the physical distance between any two points in the universe. However, as the expansion of the universe at the current local scale (for instance, planet Earth) is so small, it is not possible with the techniques available to us today to measure the laws of physics' dependency on the universe's expansion.

Very early, the Catholic Church officially proclaimed that the big bang theory is in agreement with the Bible.

# Bibliography

Aczel, Amir D. *Entanglement: The Greatest Mystery of Physics*. New York: Four Walls Eight Windows, 2002.

Badiou, Alain. *Being and Event*. New York: Bloomsbury, 2013.

Balivar, Françoise. *Einstein, Newton, Poincaré. Une histoire des principes*. Paris: Belin, 2008.

Benveniste, Émile. *Problems in General Linguistics*. Miami: University of Miami Press, 1971.

Bojowald, Martin. *Once before Time. A Whole History of the Universe*. New York: Alfred A. Kopf, 2010.

Bordelois, Yvonne. *Etimología de las pasiones*. Buenos Aires: Libros del Zorzal, 2006.

Bourdieu, Pierre. *Distinction. A Social Critique of the Judgment of Taste*. Abingdon and Oxfordshire: Routledge, 2010.

Brunschvicg, León. *Les étapes de la philosophie mathématique*. Paris: A. Blanchard, 1993.

Dawkins, Richard. *The Selfish Gene*. Oxford: Oxford University Press, 2016.

de Libera, Alain. *Archéologie du sujet, vol. 1. Naissance du sujet*. Paris: Librairie Phylosophique J. Vrin, 2007.

Derrida, Jacques. *Writing and Difference*. London and New York: Routledge and Kegan Paul, 1978.

Dodds, Eric Robertson. *The Greeks and the Irrational*. Berkeley and Los Angeles: University of California Press, 1951.

Durkheim, Émile. *The Elementary Forms of Religious Life*. Oxford: Oxford University Press, 2001.

Eidelsztein, Alfredo. "Diagnosticar el sujeto", in *Imago Agenda*, 73. Buenos Aires: Letra Viva, 2003.

Eidelsztein, Alfredo. *Las estructuras clínicas a partir de Lacan, Vol. I*. Buenos Aires: Letra Viva, 2008.

Eidelsztein, Alfredo. *The Graph of Desire. Using the Work of Jacques Lacan*. London: Karnac, 2009.

Eidelsztein, Alfredo. "La responsabilidad subjetiva," in *El Rey está desnudo*, Año 8, No. 8, 2015.

Einstein, Albert & Infeld, Leopold. *The Evolution of Physics*. New York: Simon & Schuster, 1966.

Elias, Norbert. *The Society of Individuals*. New York and London: Continuum, 1991.

Fisher, Seymour & Greenberg, Roger P. *The Limits of Biological Treatments for Psychological Distress. Comparisons with Psychotherapy and Placebo*. New York: Routledge, 2016.

Foucault, Michel. *History of Sexuality, I. The Will to Power*. New York: Pantheon Book, 1978.

Freud, Sigmund. "Psychical (or Mental) Treatment" (1890), in *Standard Edition*, Vol. VII. (London: Hogarth Press, 1953–1974).

Freud, Sigmund. "Sexuality in the Etiology of Neurosis" (1898), in *Standard Edition*, Vol. III.

Freud, Sigmund. "Fragments of the Analysis of a Case of Hysteria" (1905), in *Standard Edition*, Vol. VII.

Freud, Sigmund. "Analysis of a Phobia in Five-year-old Boy" (1909), in *Standard Edition*, Vol. X.

Freud, Sigmund. "Totem and Taboo" (1912–1913), in *Standard Edition*, Vol. XIII.

Freud, Sigmund. "From the History of an Infantile Neurosis" (1918) in *Standard Edition*, Vol. XVII.

Freud, Sigmund. "Some Additional Notes on Dream-Interpretation as a Whole" (1925), in *Standard Edition*, Vol. XIX.

Freud, Sigmund. "The Question of Lay Analysis" (1926), in *Standard Edition*, Vol. XX.

Gamow, George. *Biography of Physics*. New York: Harper, 1964.

Gangui, Alejandro. *El big bang. La génesis de nuestra cosmología*. Buenos Aires: EUDEBA, 2010.

Gárate, Ignacio & Marinas, José Miguel. *Lacan en español*. Madrid: Biblioteca Nueva, 2003.

Gimbutas, Marija. *The Language of the Goddess*. New York: Harper, 1991.

Greene, Brian. *The Fabric of the Cosmos. Space, Time, and the Texture of Reality*. New York: Alfred Knopf, 2004.

Grijelmo, Alex. *La seducción de las palabras: un recorrido por las manipulaciones del pensamiento*. Madrid: Taurus, 2000.

Hawking, Stephen W. *A Brief History of Time. From the big bang to Black Holes*. New York: Random House, 2011.

Hawking, Stephen W. & Mlodinow, Leopold. *The Grand Design*. New York: Random House, 2010.

Hurtado González, Silvia. "Los periodistas y la lengua," in *Estudios sobre el mensaje periodístico*, issue #7, pp. 295–302.

Kapuściński, Ryszard. *Travels with Herodotus*. New York: Knopf, 2009.

Kemplerer, Viktor. *Language of the Third Reich. LTI. Lingua Tertii Imperii*. New York and London: Bloomsbury, 2013.

Lacan, Jacques. *Écrits*. New York: Norton, 2006.

Lacan, Jacques. "Of Structure as an Inmixing of an Otherness Prerequisite to Any Subject Whatever," in Macksey, Richard & Donato, Eugenio (eds.), *The Structuralist Controversy. The Languages of Criticism and the Sciences of Man*. Baltimore, MD and London: The John Hopkins University Press, 1979.

Lacan, Jacques. *Seminar II*. Cambridge: UP/Norton, 1988.

Lacan, Jacques. *Seminar III*. New York: Routledge/Norton, 1993.

Lacan, Jacques. *Seminar IV*. New York: Polity, 2022.

Lacan, Jacques. *Seminar VI*. Available on www.staferla.free.fr

Lacan, Jacques. *Seminar VII*. New York: Routledge/Norton, 1992.

Lacan, Jacques. *Seminar IX*. Available on www.staferla.free.fr

Lacan, Jacques. *Seminar X*. New York: Polity, 2014.

Lacan, Jacques. *Seminar XI*. New York and London: Norton, 1981.

Lacan, Jacques. *Seminar XII*. Available on www.staferla.free.fr

Lacan, Jacques. *Seminar XIII*. Available on www.staferla.free.fr

Lacan, Jacques. *Seminar XIV*. Available on www.staferla.free.fr

Lacan, Jacques. *Seminar XVI*. Available on www.staferla.free.fr

Lacan, Jacques. *Seminar XVII.* New York: Norton, 2007.

Lacan, Jacques. *Seminar XIX.* Available on www.staferla.free.fr

Lacan, Jacques. *Seminar XX.* New York: Norton, 1998.

Lacan, Jacques. *Seminar XXI.* Available on www.staferla.free.fr

Lacan, Jacques. *Seminar XXIII.* Available on www.staferla.free.fr

Lacan, Jacques. *Seminar XXIV.* Available on www.staferla.free.fr

Lacan, Jacques. *Escansión 1.* Buenos Aires: Paidós, 1984.

Lacan, Jacques. *Intervenciones y Textos 2.* Buenos Aires: Manantial, 1988.

Lacan, Jacques. *Psicoanálisis, Radiofonía y Televisión.* Buenos Aires: Anagrama, 1977.

Mauss, Marcel. "Les techniques du corps," in Crary, Jonathan & Kwinter, Sanford (eds.), *Incorporations.* New York: Zone, 1992, pp. 455–477.

Meillassoux, Quentin. *Après la finitude. Essai sur la nécessité de la contingence.* Paris: du Seuil, 2006.

Miller, Jacques-Alain. *El Otro que no existe y sus comités de ética.* Buenos Aires, Barcelona and México: Paidós, 2005.

Miller, Jacques-Alain. *Incidencias de la última enseñanza de Lacan en la práctica analítica.* Buenos Aires: Grama, 2006.

Montesano, Haydée. "Psicoanálisis y biopolítica. 3ra. parte: Rechazo de la posición teórica que hace equivaler *jouissance* a goce. (Bio) política de una traducción," en *El rey está desnudo,* Año 3, No.4, 2011.

Morris, David B. *The Culture of Pain.* Berkeley, Los Angeles and London: University of California Press, 1991.

*Pas-tout Lacan.* Available on www.ecolelacanienne.net.

Peter, Patrick & Gangui, Alejandro. *Des défauts dans l'Univers.* Paris: CNRS, 2003.

Pinker, Stephen. *The Language Instinct. How the Mind Creates Language.* New York: W. Morrow & Co., 1994.

Pommier, Gérard. *Cómo las neurociencias demuestran el psicoanálisis.* Buenos Aires: Letra Viva, 2010.

Reichenbach, Hans. *From Copernicus to Einstein.* Berkeley, Los Angeles and London: University of California Press, 1951.

Reichenbach, Hans. *The Rise of Scientific Philosophy.* Berkeley, Los Angeles and London: University of California Press, 1951.

Reichenbach, Hans. *The Direction of Time.* Mineola, NY: Dover, 1999.

Rey, Alain, Robert, Paul & Rey-Debove, Josette. *Le grand Robert de la Langue Française.* Paris: Aubin Imprimeur, 2008.

Rosenblum, Bruce & Kuttner, Fred. *Quantum Enigma. Physics Encounter Consciousness.* New York: Oxford University Press, 2010.

Stegmüller, Wolfgang. *Teoría y experiencia.* Barcelona: Ariel, 1979.

*Unidos por la lengua. Juventud y madurez,* online resource: www.celtiberia.net (last access: May 14th, 2023).

Vázquez–Ayora, Gerardo. *Introducción a la traductología.* Washington, DC: Georgetown University School of Languages and Linguistics, 1977.

Voltaire. "Dictionnaire philosophique," in *Œuvres complètes, Section 1.* Available on www.voltaireintegral.com/19/langues.htm (last access: May 14th, 2023).

Weil, Dominique (ed.). *Homme et sujet: la subjectivité en question dans les sciences humaines.* Paris: Editions L'Harmattan, 1993.

Wilson, Edmund. *Sociobiology. The New Synthesis.* Cambridge, MA, and London: Belknap Press, 1975.

# Index

Note: Page numbers followed by "n" denote endnotes.